On Rounds:
1000 Internal
Medicine Pearls

Clinical Aphorisms *and Related* Pathophysiology

On Rounds: 1000 Internal Medicine Pearls

Clinical Aphorisms and Related Pathophysiology

Lewis Landsberg, MD

Irving S. Cutter Professor
Dean Emeritus
Northwestern University
Feinberg School of Medicine
Chicago, IL

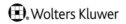

. Wolters Kluwer

Philadelphia · Baltimore · New York · London
Buenos Aires · Hong Kong · Sydney · Tokyo

Executive Editor: Rebecca Gaertner
Senior Product Development Editor: Kristina Oberle
Production Project Manager: Bridgett Dougherty
Marketing Manager: Stephanie Kindlick
Design Coordinator: Joan Wendt
Senior Manufacturing Coordinator: Beth Welsh
Prepress Vendor: Aptara, Inc.

9 8 7 6 5 4 3 2 1

Printed in China

978-1-49632-221-0
Library of Congress Cataloging-in-Publication Data
available upon request

Dedication

To my wife Jill, without whom this book would not have been written; to my students, residents, and young colleagues at Yale, Harvard, and Northwestern who have taught me more than they could ever imagine; and to my intern group at Yale, whose friendship has been a lifelong treasure.

ACKNOWLEDGMENTS

Of the many mentors who have shaped my career I would like to specifically acknowledge Paul B. Beeson, Franklin H. Epstein, Philip K. Bondy, Eugene Braunwald, and Julius Axelrod. Each of these men served as a beacon, a shining example of the clinician/scientist that I have strived, imperfectly, to emulate.

I thank Ms. Linda Carey for her skillful assistance and meticulous attention to detail in the preparation of this manuscript and for her unfailing good cheer.

Special thanks to Ms. Rebecca Gaertner at LWW for her encouragement and sound advice that contributed importantly to the final form of this book. And special thanks as well to Ms. Kristina Oberle at LWW for her expert editorial assistance and excellent taste in formatting the manuscript. Having said that, I alone bear responsibility for any errors that found their way into this book.

Finally, I thank my daughter Alison, for invaluable advice about academic publishing, and my son Judd for many fruitful discussions about congestive heart failure, extracellular fluid balance, and pulmonary function, and both of them and their spouses for Eli, Leah, Maya, Lucas, and Jonah.

PREFACE

This monograph is a compilation of aphorisms that I have found useful in almost half a century of clinical experience in internal medicine. They are the distillation of my interest in the clinical manifestations and the pathophysiology of disease. In many instances the aphorisms are derived from my own clinical observations; in some cases they reflect the experience and wisdom of others that I have come to appreciate and value over the years. In every case the aphorisms cited here, which I refer to by the time-honored designation as "pearls," have met the test of veracity and usefulness in my own clinical experience.

While no "pearl" is applicable one hundred percent of the time, I believe, nonetheless, that the ready recall of pithy statements of fact are useful aids to prompt diagnosis and treatment. Clinical medicine is filled with uncertainty, and pearls, these nuggets of accumulated wisdom, frequently simplify complicated situations and are therefore useful to both physicians in training and physicians in practice. In one sense these aphorisms represent the information store that experienced clinicians can readily bring to bear on a clinical problem. A large repertory of facts is a distinguishing feature of "master" clinicians, and an important resource of highly regarded clinical teachers.

The "pearls," indicated in bold face, are organized by organ systems for ease of reference. There is no attempt for the coverage to be comprehensive. This is not a textbook of medicine. The content reflects my own interests and experience. I have paid particular attention to those areas that, in my experience, have been a source of confusion for students and trainees.

I have also presented relevant physiology where knowledge of the underlying mechanisms improves understanding of disease pathogenesis and aids in retention of the pearls. Integrative physiology is less well taught now than previously and I believe some of the material presented here may address that deficiency.

Also included are a few "*faux pearls*" – statements that, although widely believed – are demonstrably false.

This monograph is intended for students of internal medicine. I mean students in the broad sense to include not only medical students and residents but also mature clinicians who can think about these aphorisms and the underlying physiology in relation to their own clinical experience. This book can also serve as a scaffold for the organization and augmentation of an already existing clinical data base. It should be of particular value to those clinicians that teach medical students and residents.

CONTENTS

The Clinical Evaluation

HISTORY

History of Present Illness (HPI)

The HPI is the key to the diagnosis, starting with the chief complaint. The clinical evaluation (history plus physical examination) guides the selection of tests, which are obtained to confirm or rule out diagnoses suggested clinically, an aphorism widely known as "Sutton's law."

Willie Sutton, a legendary bank robber, escaped from prison three times and always returned to bank robbing. When asked why he robbed banks he gave what has become an iconic reply: "...because that's where the money is."

The HPI orients the clinician to the patient's problem and establishes an initial differential diagnosis. Of major importance is the temporal sequence and progression of symptoms.

Elements from the Review of Systems and the Past Medical History that are relevant to the patient's complaint should be part of the HPI. Pertinent negatives should be enumerated. If not specifically stated, a negative cannot be inferred; it must be presumed that the question was not asked.

Symptoms that have a limited differential are particularly important.

Paroxysmal nocturnal dyspnea (PND), when classic, means left heart failure; by contrast, orthopnea has an extensive differential and is much less specific although it is also a manifestation of heart failure.

This distinction is only meaningful when the features of PND are known and understood: awakening from asleep after about 2 hours (usually around 2 AM)

1

with shortness of breath, getting out of bed, and sitting in a chair, usually for the rest of the night.

PND results from the gradual redistribution of fluid, accumulated in the periphery (lower extremities) during the day, to the central compartment where the ensuing volume load exceeds the output capacity of the compromised myocardium raising the end diastolic pressure of the left ventricle. By contrast, in a variety of diseases breathing is made easier upright than supine (orthopnea) and the discomfort is felt immediately on lying down.

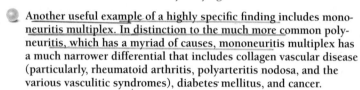 Another useful example of a highly specific finding includes mononeuritis multiplex. In distinction to the much more common polyneuritis, which has a myriad of causes, mononeuritis multiplex has a much narrower differential that includes collagen vascular disease (particularly, rheumatoid arthritis, polyarteritis nodosa, and the various vasculitic syndromes), diabetes mellitus, and cancer.

Pain

Pain is a frequent presenting complaint for many diseases. The history provides important diagnostic clues about the origin of pain.

Pain that is aggravated by movement, and that makes the patient lie still is characteristic of an inflammatory process.

The patient's reaction to pain is more important than the subjective descriptions of the pain itself.

With an acute inflammatory abdominal process like cholecystitis or pancreatitis the patient lies absolutely still.

Colic, pain that waxes and wanes, indicates pressure changes in a hollow viscus such as the biliary system or ureter; it is brought on by obstruction, usually from a stone. The response to colicky pain is characterized by an inability to get comfortable and by writhing around or pacing the floor.

Maneuvers that accentuate or ameliorate the pain are also important to note.

Pleuritic chest pain, for example, is worsened by deep breathing or coughing, reflecting inflammation of the parietal pleura.

THE PHYSICAL EXAMINATION

To become expert at physical examination requires practice. Establishing the bounds of normality, and therefore the ability to elicit the abnormal finding when present, requires experience and attention to detail.

Although advanced imaging and other testing have unfortunately and inappropriately denigrated the value of physical examination (PE), it remains the cornerstone of clinical evaluation for the following reasons.

1. It is virtually harmless, distinguishing it from many other modes of evaluation.
2. Along with the history it guides all subsequent investigations.
3. It is neither feasible nor desirable to do widespread testing without a clinical evaluation first. When prior probability of a disease is low, false-positive tests abound.
4. It is useful for assessing progression of disease and response to treatment.
5. The "laying on of hands" strengthens the physician–patient relationship.

When encountering a new patient with an undiagnosed disease a full examination should be performed and all organ systems assessed even while concentrating on the area suggested by the history. A full examination includes noting and describing the attitude of the patient in bed and a careful recording of the vital signs. In addition to listening to the chest and palpating the abdomen, feeling for all pulses, testing strength in all major muscle groups, eliciting and recording all reflexes, assessing the cranial nerves, and (with some exceptions) a genital and rectal examination should be part of every physical.

In a patient with leg pain, for example, how will you be certain of an absent pedal pulse if you have not examined this in many patients without lower extremity vascular disease? In assessing the likelihood of increased intracranial pressure how will you identify papilledema if you have not examined many normal fundi and noted the presence (or absence) of venous pulsations?

LABORATORY TESTS

Never let a single laboratory result dissuade you from a diagnosis strongly suggested by the weight of the clinical findings.

Discordant laboratory results should be repeated.

Always start with the least specialized tests. A CBC is always indicated in the evaluation of a sick patient where the diagnosis is not known. The CBC contains a lot of information, much of which is frequently overlooked.

A WBC without a differential is not interpretable and therefore useless.

The percentage of polymorphonuclear leukocytes (granulocytes) and the presence of immature forms (bands), in comparison to the percentage of mononuclear cells (lymphocytes plus monocytes) are of particular importance.

The presence of eosinophils argues forcefully against bacterial infection.

In the absence of a documented pre-existing cause for eosinophilia the usual mediators of inflammation and the hormonal response to severe illness effectively clear the blood of eosinophils.

Toxic granulation, an outpouring of immature granulocytes with large granules and vacuoles, indicates infection.

An elevated platelet count is a very good marker of an inflammatory process.

An elevated sedimentation rate (ESR) is unlikely to be helpful except in cases of temporal arteritis or subacute thyroiditis, where very high values are the rule.

ESR may be normal in the face of significant inflammation and modest elevations are too nonspecific to be useful.

ESR may, however, be elevated in dysproteinemias where the paraprotein causes clumping of the red cells or rouleaux formation.

Examination of the blood smear, therefore, may provide useful clues to the diagnosis.

IMAGING

Usefulness of the Chest X-ray

Although modern imaging techniques and sophisticated computer software have revolutionized diagnosis (as described in specific situations throughout this book), it is surprising that the simple chest x-ray still provides much useful information.

Although much less frequently used now than in the past, the PA and lateral chest x-ray can provide much useful information. Portable AP films are much less helpful.

There is no substitute for personally reviewing the chest x-ray.

Specific cardiac chamber enlargement can be assessed from the lateral view.

The right ventricle comprises the anterior border of the cardiac silhouette in the lateral view. Normally, the right ventricle abuts the sternum one-third of the way up and on a very steep angle; with right ventricular hypertrophy the cardiac silhouette hits the sternum one-half way up, the retrosternal space is diminished, and the angle is no longer acute (one could stand on it without falling off!). The posterior border of the heart in the lateral view is made up of the left ventricle. With left ventricular hypertrophy the retrocardiac space is compromised and the angle formed with the inferior vena cava is diminished.

Calcification in the costochondral cartilage in the elderly is frequently associated with mitral annulus calcification, so the former should prompt a look for the latter.

This may be an important clue to the presence of significant mitral regurgitation.

In evaluating pneumonic infiltrates the presence or absence of air bronchograms and the effect of the infiltrate on lung volume provide significant information as to the underlying cause.

Air bronchograms without loss of volume indicate a pneumonic consolidation like pneumonia, a so-called alveolar infiltrate; volume loss implies bronchial obstruction.

- **Location of the abnormality is important: upper lobe infiltrates suggest tuberculosis (TB) or fungal infection. TB is located classically in the posterior segment of the upper lobe; fungal disease in the anterior segment. Bullae are typically located in the upper lobes; middle or lower lobe bullae suggest α1-antitrypsin deficiency.**

The lateral view is also helpful in assessing hilar fullness; a dense shadow in the shape of a donut suggests hilar lymphadenopathy; pulmonary vessels appear much less dense.

- **When the left hemidiaphragm is higher than the right, the possibility of a subdiaphragmatic process (abscess, enlarged spleen, adrenal mass) should be considered.**

The right hemidiaphragm is normally higher than the left because it sits on the liver below.

- **Inability to "take a deep breath" during a chest x-ray does not reflect an inadequate attempt by the patient.**

There is usually an underlying cause such as pain (in the chest or abdomen), muscle weakness, or congestive heart failure. In the latter excess fluid in the lung parenchyma decreases compliance and restricts the ability to "take a deep breath." It is a *faux pearl* that the diminished diaphragmatic excursion reflects "poor inspiratory effort."

SOME WIDELY APPLICABLE CLINICAL APHORISMS

Occam's Razor: The Law of Parsimony as Applied to Diagnosis

- **Patients frequently present with constellations of symptoms and signs that may appear unrelated; in general, the best diagnosis will encompass an explanation that accounts for all the findings.**

Occam's razor cuts best in younger patients. In the elderly, the coincidental occurrence of several diseases will often contribute to the clinical picture.

- **The experienced clinician will quickly identify the few crucial findings in a complicated case that must be explained by the diagnosis.**

These will often lead to an appropriate differential and point to the correct diagnosis.

- **The final diagnosis must explain the chief complaint.**

Therapeutics

 You can't make an asymptomatic patient feel better. ("Never shoot a singing bird.")

Related old adages include: *primum non nocere* (firstly do no harm); less is frequently more in the elderly. Loeb's first and second laws state the obvious: if a patient improves during a course of treatment, continue it; if a patient worsens under treatment, stop it. (Robert Loeb was a renowned professor of medicine at Columbia.) Loeb's third law has been banned in the interests of professionalism ("never trust a surgeon").

Blood 2

T he cellular elements of blood, although subject to specific diseases in their own right, are affected in most diseases of other organ systems as well, and in many of these the changes in the blood contribute to the pathogenesis, the symptomatology, and the complications of the underlying disease. This is reflected by the inclusion of a wide variety of topics in this section. Topics that frequently cause confusion or are poorly understood are dealt with in some detail.

ANEMIA

Loss of oxygen-carrying capacity of the blood results in a myriad of nonspecific but well-known symptoms such as fatigue, headache and listlessness, and tachycardia. Pale skin and conjunctival pallor are obvious signs.

When the hemoglobin (Hgb) falls below 4 g/dL the palmar creases lose their pink color, a hallmark of severe anemia.

● Shortness of breath is an underappreciated manifestation of moderate to severe anemia, reflecting insufficient tissue oxygenation.

● In organ systems where the circulation is compromised from underlying vascular disease, anemia may precipitate dramatic symptoms, resulting in decompensation of a previously marginally compensated state. This is particularly true for the cerebral and the coronary circulations.

Thus in patients with underlying coronary artery disease (CAD), angina or myocardial infarction (MI) may occur, and marginally compensated heart failure may become full blown; more dramatically, in the presence of asymptomatic cerebrovascular disease, a complete hemiparesis may develop which reverts with transfusion and restoration of oxygenation.

Characterization of the Anemia

Red cell indices, developed by Wintrobe in the 1920s, have provided the basis for the classification of anemic states since that time. They provide a measure of the size (MCV) and the Hgb content (MCH and MCHC) of the red cells.

Microcytic Anemias

Hypochromic microcytic anemia (low MCV and low MCH) indicates iron deficiency or hemoglobinopathy; RBCs are pale on smear.

● Anemia with a low MCV in a man means blood loss (iron deficiency) and necessitates a gastrointestinal (GI) workup.

An exception is in thalassemia minor where the MCV is very low and the smear is very abnormal.

● Celiac sprue may also cause iron deficiency without bleeding.

● Unusually heavy menses frequently causes iron deficiency in women. The new onset of increased menstrual flow should raise the possibility of thrombocytopenia.

● Hypothyroidism is another cause of heavy menstrual bleeding.

● Iron deficiency anemia, especially in women and children, may be associated with pagophagia, a peculiar pica for ice.

A history of eating ice cubes should be a tipoff to an underlying iron deficiency anemia. The mechanism is obscure, but the pica resolves after appropriate treatment with iron.

Hemolytic Anemias

Many different processes may result in RBC destruction: mechanical factors, immune-mediated processes, pharmaceuticals, and genetic or acquired alterations in RBC membranes. Evidence of hemolysis includes a rise in indirect bilirubin; a low serum haptoglobin, increased plasma lactic acid dehydrogenase (LDH), and spherocytes on the peripheral smear.

> Rapid turnover of red cell precursors in the marrow of patients with hemolytic anemia may be associated with folate deficiency.

Folate replacement, therefore, is part of the treatment of hemolytic anemias.

Microangiopathic Hemolytic Anemia

> Schistocytes and helmet cells indicate a microangiopathic process which has a limited differential and is therefore useful diagnostically. The differential includes thrombotic thrombocytopenic purpura (TTP), disseminated intravascular coagulation (DIC), and malignant hypertension. Malignancy also may cause microangiopathic hemolysis (most commonly with mucinous adenocarcinomas); DIC is the likely cause of the association of microangiopathic hemolytic anemia with cancer.

The microangiopathy is caused by activation of the coagulation cascade with fibrin deposition and stranding in small arterioles; these fibrin strands sheer the red cells and damage platelets as they pass through the circulation. In malignant hypertension fibrinoid necrosis in the arterioles is the inciting event that leads to fibrin deposition. Anything that produces widespread endothelial injury may initiate the process including pharmaceuticals, and infectious agents.

> Red cell damage also occurs with dysfunctional cardiac valves, usually artificial or heavily calcified valves, which beat up the red cells (the so-called "Waring Blender" syndrome), thereby causing hemolysis.

Autoimmune Hemolytic Anemia

> Autoimmune hemolytic anemia with positive direct Coombs test occurs with lymphoproliferative diseases and with collagen vascular disease, most notably systemic lupus erythematosus (SLE).

In acquired autoimmune hemolytic anemia the patients' autoantibodies interact with RBC components; the affected RBCs are cleared in the spleen.

> Since the hemolysis in autoimmune hemolytic anemias occurs principally outside the circulation haptoglobin is reduced only slightly or not at all, despite the fact that the hemolytic process may be quite severe.

The autoantibodies are said to be "warm" in that hemolysis occurs at normal body temperature (37 °C). These consist primarily of IgG.

> The direct Coombs test detects the autoantibodies on the patients' RBCs by agglutination of the red cells when incubated with antiglobulin sera raised in animals.

The indirect Coombs test detects antibodies in the patients' sera directed to normal subjects' red cells. It is used in type and cross match and in detecting transfusion reactions.

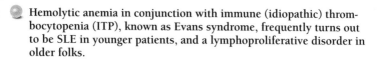

Hemolytic anemia in conjunction with immune (idiopathic) thrombocytopenia (ITP), known as Evans syndrome, frequently turns out to be SLE in younger patients, and a lymphoproliferative disorder in older folks.

Evans syndrome should provoke a workup for lupus and/or lymphocytic malignancy depending on the clinical features.

Cold agglutinins are antibodies that bind to red cells at temperatures below 37 °C; the resulting hemolysis occurs in cold exposed areas and is usually mild. Mycoplasma pneumonia and infectious mononucleosis are common infections associated with the formation of cold agglutinins.

A bedside test showing red cell clumping in an anticoagulated tube of blood when exposed to ice water makes a nice demonstration. The autoantibodies are IgM.

Hemolytic anemia with leukopenia, thrombocytopenia, and venous thrombosis is highly suggestive of paroxysmal nocturnal hemoglobinuria (PNH).

This rare disorder is caused by acquired hematopoietic stem cell surface protein deficiencies that render the cells sensitive to normal levels of complement in the circulation with resultant intravascular hemolysis and hemoglobinuria.

Venous thrombosis, particularly of the intra-abdominal vessels including the portal and hepatic veins, is not uncommon in PNH and may reflect a tendency of the platelets to aggregate in the presence of complement.

Symptoms are intermittent.

The slight respiratory acidosis that occurs during sleep had been thought to trigger attacks giving rise to the "nocturnal" designation in the name of the disease. This is probably an erroneous explanation. The fact that morning urine is heavily concentrated probably accounts for the red color noted on arising. Hemoglobinuria results from the intravascular hemolysis that occurs in this disease.

The old standby treatments included transfusions, corticosteroids, and supportive care; a newer treatment involves a monoclonal antibody attack on complement.

Drug-induced hemolytic anemias are most common with penicillin, cephalosporins, methyl dopa, quinine, and sulfonamides.

A careful drug history is part of the evaluation of hemolytic anemia.

Delayed hemolytic transfusion reactions are another cause of hemolysis that is frequently overlooked.

In persons sensitized by prior blood transfusions or pregnancy an anamnestic antibody response directed against minor RBC antigens (Kidd, Duffy, and Kell, for example) may develop days to weeks after the transfusion and cause hemolysis of the transfused blood. Such reactions are associated with extravascular hemolysis and a positive direct Coombs test which was not present during the pretransfusion cross match because the antibody was present in titers too low to detect.

Megaloblastic Anemias

Megaloblastic anemia results from a defect in red cell DNA synthesis which alters and delays RBC maturation resulting in altered ("megaloblastic") differentiation. The cause is vitamin B_{12} or folic acid deficiency; the involvement of B_{12} results from its role in folate metabolism.

Folate is required for normal DNA synthesis; inadequate availability of folate causes megaloblastic differentiation in the red cell line. The methyltetrahydrofolate trap hypothesis explains how B_{12} deficiency results in megaloblastosis by reducing folate availability for RBC maturation (Fig. 2-1).

Vitamin B_{12}, a critical cofactor for methyl group transfers, is required for the regeneration of tetrahydrofolate from methyltetrahydrofolate. Tetrahydrofolate is a form of the vitamin that can be utilized for DNA synthesis. In the absence of B_{12}, folate is trapped in the methylated form which is a metabolic dead end that cannot be utilized for RBC maturation.

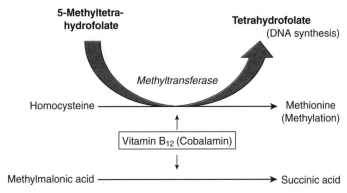

FIGURE 2.1 The methyltetrahydrofolate trap hypothesis: the relationship between folate and vitamin B_{12} in the pathogenesis of the megaloblastic anemias. Tetrahydrofolate is required for DNA synthesis. In bone marrow rapid cell turnover requires adequate supplies of tetrahydrofolate for normal cell maturation. Methyltetrahydrofolate is a metabolite involved in methyl group transfers including the synthesis of methionine from homocysteine, but is not functional in DNA synthesis. Cyanocobalamin (vitamin B_{12}) is required to regenerate the tetrahydrofolate form which is necessary for normal DNA synthesis and normal red cell maturation. In pernicious anemia (PA) the absence of B_{12} causes a deficiency of usable folate at the cellular level resulting in megaloblastic differentiation. B_{12} is also required for myelin synthesis and the conversion of methylmalonic acid to succinate; buildup of methylmalonic acid in the blood is now the preferred test for the diagnosis of PA.

In B_{12} deficiency, therefore, folate is not available for DNA synthesis, causing a functional folate deficiency at the cellular level and the development of a megaloblastic state.

- The RBCs resulting from megaloblastic differentiation are large (macro-ovalocytes) due to delayed maturation; corresponding changes in the granulocytic cell line lead to multisegmented polymorphonuclear leukocytes.

- Nonmegaloblastic macrocytosis may be seen in hypothyroidism, although it should be recognized that hypothyroidism and PA (along with other autoimmune diseases) not infrequently coexist.

Pernicious Anemia (PA)

Deficiency of vitamin B_{12} results in PA.

- PA is most common in persons of Northern European descent and is frequently associated with blue eyes, big ears, a sallow yellow complexion, and premature graying of the hair (white before 40 years of age).

Premature graying is a marker for autoimmune disease in general. The anemia (pallor) in concert with low-grade jaundice may produce a distinctive "lemon yellow" coloration of the skin.

- B_{12} deficiency is virtually never dietary in origin except in the case of severe and long-standing veganism; B_{12} deficiency results rather from a failure of the gastric mucosa to produce intrinsic factor which is essential for the normal absorption of the vitamin in the ileum.

In PA atrophic gastritis is associated with achlorhydria and failure to produce intrinsic factor.

- Ileal disease such as regional enteritis (Crohn's disease) or surgical ileal resection, total or partial gastrectomy, and blind loop syndromes are other potential causes of vitamin B_{12} deficiency.

- Intestinal motility disorders with bacterial overgrowth in the small bowel may cause B_{12} deficiency since the bacteria utilize and compete for dietary B_{12}.

Folate may be normal under intestinal overgrowth situations as folic acid is synthesized by the overgrown bacteria.

- Since the hepatic stores of B_{12} are extensive it takes years for the development of anemia to appear after B_{12} absorption is impaired.

The anemia in PA develops chronically and may be very severe with Hgb as low as 3 or 4 g/dL. This necessitates slow and cautious transfusion to avoid pulmonary edema.

● The conversion of methylmalonic acid to succinic acid is a B_{12} dependent reaction; in B_{12} deficiency methylmalonic acid builds up and elevated levels have become a standard test for PA (Fig. 2-1).

Likewise, the conversion of homocysteine to methionine requires B_{12}, so elevated levels of homocysteine are also useful in the diagnosis of PA.

● Plasma levels of B_{12} levels are much less reliable than methylmalonic levels in the diagnosis of PA.

Autoantibodies may interfere in the B_{12} assay with erroneous elevation of the B_{12} level.

● Neurologic changes develop in PA independent of the anemia and consist of demyelination in the lateral and dorsal columns of the spinal cord, resulting in impaired position sense and spasticity of the lower extremities (combined system disease).

Clinically, this results in a positive Romberg test and a positive Babinski sign. Personality change and outright dementia may occur as well.

Vitamin B_{12} is necessary for normal myelin synthesis and deficient supply of this vitamin underlies the neurologic abnormalities that occur in PA. Typical neurologic changes of PA do not occur in folate-related megaloblastic anemias, although peripheral neuropathy may be present with folic acid deficiency.

● Large doses of folic acid may bypass the methyltetrahydrofolate trap, thereby masking the hematologic changes in PA and allowing the serious neurologic consequences of B_{12} deficiency to progress.

It is also possible that excess folate obligates the diminished B_{12} stores to the heme synthesis pathway by drawing B_{12} from its role in myelin synthesis, thereby worsening the neurologic abnormalities of PA.

● Folic acid supplements should never be given to patients with megaloblastic anemia until PA has been ruled out.

Folate Deficiency

Folic acid deficiency, the other cause of megaloblastic anemia, is caused by inadequate nutrition or impaired folate absorption.

● Folate deficiency frequently occurs in association with alcoholism, and is potentiated by physiologic situations of increased demand, such as pregnancy, and in diseases with increased bone marrow turnover like the hemolytic anemias.

● Impaired absorption is also an important cause of folate deficiency. Folic acid in food is conjugated with glutamate and needs to be deconjugated before it can be absorbed.

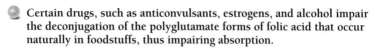

Certain drugs, such as anticonvulsants, estrogens, and alcohol impair the deconjugation of the polyglutamate forms of folic acid that occur naturally in foodstuffs, thus impairing absorption.

Folate deficiency is very common in alcoholics due to poor dietary intake and impaired absorption.

Folate supplements given orally as treatment are not in the polyglutamate form and do not require deconjugation.

Folate malabsorption is common in celiac sprue.

Hemoglobin Abnormalities

The function of Hgb to bind, store, and release oxygen depends on heme which contains iron in the reduced (ferrous) state.

The relationship between Hgb and oxygen is expressed in the Hgb–oxygen dissociation curve which represents the percentage saturation of Hgb as a function of the partial pressure of oxygen (Fig. 2-2). Physiologic factors that alter this relationship include pH, temperature, and RBC 2,3 diphosphoglycerate (2,3-DPG, also known as 2,3-BPG).

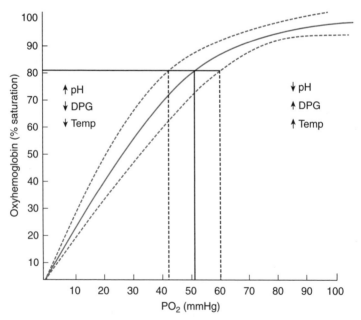

FIGURE 2.2 The oxyhemoglobin dissociation curve: relationship between oxygen saturation of hemoglobin and the partial pressure of oxygen in the blood. Factors that shift the curve to the right (acidosis, fever, and increased 2,3-DPG) enhance oxygen delivery to tissues.

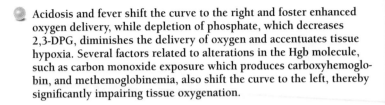 Acidosis and fever shift the curve to the right and foster enhanced oxygen delivery, while depletion of phosphate, which decreases 2,3-DPG, diminishes the delivery of oxygen and accentuates tissue hypoxia. Several factors related to alterations in the Hgb molecule, such as carbon monoxide exposure which produces carboxyhemoglobin, and methemoglobinemia, also shift the curve to the left, thereby significantly impairing tissue oxygenation.

Oxidative Damage to RBCs

RBCs are particularly vulnerable to oxidative injury since they both carry oxygen and lack cellular organelles and the full biochemical repertory that afford protection to other cells that contain nuclei and mitochondria.

Oxidative damage to the RBC can occur either by 1) disruption of the cell membrane and denaturation of the RBC proteins which form Heinz bodies or 2) by oxidation of the iron in heme from the ferrous to the ferric form resulting in methhemoglobin.

Distinct clinical syndromes result from each form of damage, and distinct intracellular mechanisms exist to counter the effects of oxidation on RBC proteins and RBC heme respectively.

An elaborate system protects RBC proteins and membranes from oxidative damage by utilizing the pentose phosphate shunt which generates reduced NADP-H; the latter drives the regeneration of glutathione from its oxidized disulfide state. The glutathione thus formed is the major antioxidant in the red cell which protects RBC proteins and membranes from oxidative damage.

Insufficient reserves of glutathione results in denaturation of the RBC proteins which clump and attach to the RBC membrane, thus distorting the architecture and damaging the distensibility of the cell. The damaged red cells are removed by the spleen resulting in extravascular hemolysis.

The clumped denatured RBC proteins are known as Heinz bodies, visible on supra vital staining of the blood smear; the resulting hemolytic anemias are referred to as Heinz body anemias.

The altered erythrocytes are removed by the spleen (extravascular hemolysis). Removal of the Heinz bodies located at the RBC surface results in characteristic "bite cells."

The initial step in the reductive resynthesis of glutathione by the pentose phosphate shunt is the oxidation of glucose-6-phosphate catalyzed by the enzyme *glucose-6-phosphate dehydrogenase* (G6PD).

G6PD Deficiency

G6PD deficiency, an x-linked recessive trait, and the most common inherited enzyme deficiency in humans, renders the RBCs susceptible to oxidative stress, and the affected patients subject to repeated bouts of acute hemolytic anemia.

The disease is most common in patients of Middle Eastern, Mediterranean, and African descent. There is a suggestion, as with sickle cell anemia, that G6PD deficiency may afford protection from malaria, accounting for the persistence of the trait over the course of evolution. Many different mutations have been noted and the severity of the enzyme deficiency depends on the particular mutation. African American males have a mutation associated with more severe disease.

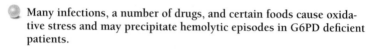 **Many infections, a number of drugs, and certain foods cause oxidative stress and may precipitate hemolytic episodes in G6PD deficient patients.**

Although unproven, phagocytosis associated with infections may release oxidants that precipitate attacks. Antimalarials, sulfa drugs, and some antibiotics are the common agents in provoking hemolysis. Fava beans are the classic food that induces attacks. The disease in the Middle East and Mediterranean areas was historically noted as "Favism."

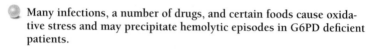 **The oldest RBCs have the lowest levels of G6PD and are hemolyzed preferentially. This limits the length of each acute episode which ends when the most vulnerable cells have been destroyed.**

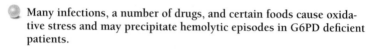 **Assaying for G6PD activity during an acute attack may fail to demonstrate enzyme deficiency since the young RBCs remaining after the older ones are destroyed have sufficient enzymatic activity to yield a false positive result.**

Methemoglobinemia

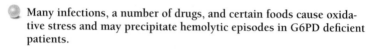 **Methemoglobin contains iron in the oxidized ferric form rendering it unable to bind oxygen while simultaneously shifting the Hgb–oxygen dissociation curve of the unoxidized ferrous heme to the left. The net result is failure of the RBCs to release oxygen to metabolizing tissues causing tissue hypoxia despite normal PaO_2, and turning the color of blood a dark brown.**

Auto-oxidation of the ferrous ion in heme to the ferric state occurs continuously at a low rate; the ferric ion thus formed is reduced to the ferrous state by an RBC reductase enzyme that utilizes NADH. This limits the level of methemoglobin to less than 1% of the total Hgb concentration. Congenital methemoglobinemia is due to inborn deficiency of the reductase; the more common acquired form is due to drug-induced oxidation of the ferrous ion.

Note that the glutathione reducing system utilizes NAD**P**-H which cannot convert the ferric ion to the ferrous form.

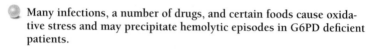 **Local anesthetics, Dapsone, and nitrous oxide are common causes of acquired methemoglobinemia.**

Acute methemoglobinemia during endoscopic procedures may develop as a consequence of using benzocaine or other local anesthetics

 Methylene blue is used therapeutically to reduce the ferric ion in heme to the ferrous state.

Under normal physiologic conditions the glutathione reductive pathway cannot reduce the ferric ion to the ferrous state due to the absence, in RBCs, of an electron acceptor for NADPH. Methylene blue provides such an acceptor enabling the glutathione system to reduce the ferric iron and regenerate normal ferrous heme. Note, however, that methylene blue should never be given to patients with G6PD deficiency.

Hemoglobinopathies

Sickle cell anemia, the first disease to be understood in molecular terms, results in clumping of desaturated Hgb, deformation of the affected RBCs, sludging of blood, and occlusion of small vessels resulting in tissue ischemia, manifested clinically as painful crises. Shortened red cell survival leads to anemia. Carriers of the sickle trait (S/A hemoglobin–heterozygote for the S gene) are generally not anemic and do not suffer crises.

 Unexplained bouts of hematuria in young African Americans are usually caused by sickle trait.

In individuals with sickle trait RBC sickling does occur in the renal medulla since this area of the kidney is relatively anoxic, and has a high osmolality, both factors which are known to potentiate sickling in S/A RBCs. Arteriolar occlusion is the result with ischemia of the renal medulla leading to papillary necrosis. This usually occurs in adolescence or young adult life, may be clinically silent, or may cause bouts of unexplained hematuria, or renal colic from the sloughed papilla. Isosthenuria with polyuria is the eventual consequence in all patients with sickle trait.

 An abundance of target cells in the peripheral smear is highly suggestive of Hgb C or SC disease.

 Familial cases of polycythemia should raise the suspicion of Hgb variants with increased affinity for oxygen.

Rare Hgb variants have a tighter than normal affinity for oxygen (Hgb –oxygen dissociation curve shifted to the left) with consequent tissue hypoxia and a compensatory increase in RBC production. These unusual variants are a rare cause of polycythemia, frequently occurring in families.

Normochromic–Normocytic Anemia

A wide variety of diseases are associated with normochromic–normocytic red cell morphology.

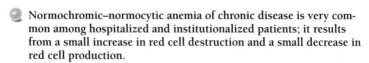

Normochromic–normocytic anemia of chronic disease is very common among hospitalized and institutionalized patients; it results from a small increase in red cell destruction and a small decrease in red cell production.

These changes usually reflect an underlying inflammatory process with associated cytokine production. Diagnostic workup fails to identify a hematologic cause.

Pure red cell aplasia, aplastic anemia, myelodysplastic syndromes, myelopthisis, and myelofibrosis are all associated with anemia that is usually normochromic–normocytic but may be microcytic.

The blood smear in these diseases is frequently abnormal with prominent anisocytosis. Examination of the bone marrow is essential for diagnosis and the findings reflect the underlying cause. Frequently the cause is unknown, but in some cases toxin exposure (solvents, particularly benzene), specific infections, or malignancy may be implicated.

PLATELETS

Thrombocytopenia and Purpura

There are many causes of thrombocytopenia: viral infections, auto-immune destruction, drugs, alcohol, folate deficiency, peripheral consumption (DIC), marrow failure, hypersplenism, cancer chemotherapy, and hematologic malignancies.

A platelet count below 20,000 μL may be associated with serious bleeding in response to trauma; spontaneous (life-threatening) hemorrhage may occur at counts below 10,000; counts below 50,000 may cause bleeding in response to minor trauma.

Deficiency of platelets prolongs the bleeding time, tends to be superficial involving the skin and mucous membranes, and occurs promptly after trauma. Menorrhagia is a common manifestation. Petechiae are often the earliest manifestation, coalescing into purpura.

Very low platelet counts may be associated with dangerous central nervous system (CNS) or GI bleeding.

In distinction to thrombocytopenia, abnormalities of the clotting cascade, such as classic hemophilia, cause deep bleeding into joints (hemarthroses), muscles, and viscera.

In clotting factor deficiency diseases the whole blood clotting time, and plasma measures of coagulation (partial thromboplastin time [PTT]), are prolonged and bleeding occurs hours after trauma, rather than immediately, since platelets provide the initial hemostatic mechanism.

Petechiae are small, nonblanching, nonpalpable reddish macules most common on the lower extremities where the hydrostatic forces are greatest. Palpable petechiae occur with vasculitis.

In contrast, pink morbilliform rashes like those occurring with viral exanthems or drug reactions, blanch with applied pressure.

- A wide variety of common viral infections cause mild thrombocytopenia not associated with bleeding. Usually unnoticed, no treatment or evaluation is necessary. More prolonged or profound thrombocytopenia may occur with human immunodeficiency virus (HIV), hepatitis C virus (HCV), Epstein-Barr virus (EBV), and rickettsial diseases.

The peripheral blood smear must be inspected in every case of thrombocytopenia to ascertain the presence or absence of microangiopathic changes.

- Shistocytes and helmet cells are characteristic of microangiopathy and suggest the diagnosis of TTP.

The presence or absence of these changes helps identify the underlying cause of the thrombocytopenia and leads to specific therapy: plasmapheresis or intravenous gamma globulin (IVG) for TTP, steroids for ITP.

Idiopathic Thrombocytopenic Purpura (ITP)

The clinical manifestation of ITP is the appearance of petechiae, especially on the lower extremities where they may coalesce into purpuric blotches.

- Also called immune thrombocytopenia, ITP is caused by an autoantibody (IgG) directed against platelet glycoproteins; the tagged platelets are then removed from the circulation by the reticuloendothelial system.

- The antiplatelet antibodies in ITP may or may not be detected by available clinical assays, so their absence does not rule out ITP.

- The diagnosis of ITP depends on ruling out other causes of thrombocytopenia.

Since the thrombocytopenia is caused by peripheral destruction, bone marrow aspirate reveals increased megakaryocytes.

- ITP may be triggered by an antecedent infection, especially in children.

Prognosis for remission with or without immunosuppression is better in children than in adults.

Thrombotic Thrombocytopenic Purpura (TTP)

- TTP is caused by microvascular thrombi in multiple organs that result in a classic pentad of symptoms and signs: thrombocytopenic purpura, microangiopathic hemolytic anemia, neurologic manifestations, fever, and decreased renal function.

The cause is deficiency of a metalloproteinase that breaks down large aggregates of von Willebrand factor (vWF). The resulting vWF multimers cause platelet clumping and initiate the thrombotic process. The enzyme deficiency may be congenital, but is usually acquired and results from an autoantibody to the enzyme responsible for cleaving the vWF multimers.

Plasmapheresis has dramatically altered the outlook for this disease which was invariably fatal before the benefit of exchange transfusion was recognized.

> **Hemolytic-uremic syndrome (HUS) is a related disease mostly of children that usually follows an episode of infectious diarrhea.**

Renal failure is more prominent in HUS than in TTP and CNS symptoms less common. *Shiga* toxin-producing *Escherichia coli* O157:H7 is the classic, but by no means the exclusive, cause.

Disseminated Intravascular Coagulation (DIC)

> **Also known as a consumptive coagulopathy, DIC occurs when the coagulation cascade is inappropriately activated in response to severe infection, malignancy, trauma, toxins, or obstetric emergencies.**

Uncontrolled intravascular coagulation triggered by exposure of the blood to the procoagulant "tissue factor" and consequent fibrinolysis consume the components of the coagulation system resulting in the paradoxical combination of bleeding and thrombi-induced organ ischemia.

> **Thrombocytopenia, prolonged prothrombin time (PT), and prolonged PTT are characteristics of DIC and useful in diagnosis.**

Fibrinogen, which is also consumed in DIC, may or may not be low since it may be elevated as an acute phase reactant in many of the situations in which DIC occurs.

> **Fibrin split products (FSPs) and D-dimer are elevated in DIC as a consequence of fibrinolysis.**

> **Malignancy-associated DIC occurs most commonly with promyelocytic leukemia and mucinous adenocarcinomas.**

Drug-induced Thrombocytopenias

Aside from chemotherapeutic or immunosuppressive drugs, which affect bone marrow platelet development and have thrombocytopenia as an expected consequence of therapy, many pharmaceuticals cause the peripheral destruction of platelets by an immune mechanism.

> **The most common causes of drug-induced thrombocytopenia include heparin, quinidine and quinine, the penicillins, and thiazide diuretics. Of these, heparin is the most common, the most severe, and thus the most important cause.**

There are two types of heparin-induced thrombocytopenia (HIT): Type I, the more common type results from an interaction of heparin with platelets that causes platelet clumping and modest reduction of the platelet count. It is self-limited, begins within 2 days of the initiation of heparin and is not associated with bleeding or thrombotic complications.

🔵 **Type II HIT is an immune-mediated reaction in which heparin interacts with platelets, stimulates an antibody against the heparin platelet complex, resulting ultimately in platelet aggregation and endothelial damage. Despite the thrombocytopenia, it is thrombosis, and not hemorrhage, that results and causes the morbidity.**

Type II HIT is a potentially severe reaction that typically begins after 4 days of heparin administration. The resulting thrombotic events affect the venous and, less commonly, the arterial circulations. The designation HIT, if unmodified, refers to the type II reaction.

🔵 **HIT may be induced by minimal heparin exposure such as that occurring with IV flushes. The reaction is much less common (but does occur) with low molecular weight heparins than with the unfractionated compound.**

Treatment, in addition to immediate cessation of all heparin products, involves direct or indirect thrombin inhibitors (not warfarin until the platelet count normalizes). This is essential in all patients since the risk of thrombosis is ongoing for at least 2 to 3 months.

🔵 **After an episode of HIT heparin is to be avoided for life.**

Other Causes of Petechiae and Purpura

🔵 **Petechiae and purpura may also occur with normal platelet counts and normal platelet function. In these cases, vasculitis, capillary fragility, or capillary damage from infection or toxins may be involved.**

Henoch–Schönlein purpura, autoerythrocyte sensitization, senile purpura, and scurvy are a few examples.

🔵 **Henoch–Schönlein purpura, more common in children but also occurring in adults, is an IgA and complement-mediated vasculitis, in which the petechiae are palpable and the platelet count normal or elevated.**

Arthritis of the large joints and abdominal pain are usually associated.

🔵 **Autoerythrocyte sensitization, an obscure and poorly understood entity usually affecting young women, consists of recurrent attacks of painful purpura and ecchymoses involving predominantly the legs. All coagulation studies in these patients are normal.**

Also known as psychogenic purpura or the Gardner–Diamond syndrome, the attacks may be precipitated by stress and frequently occur in women with emotional problems. The purpura can be reproduced by the subcutaneous injection of RBC stroma.

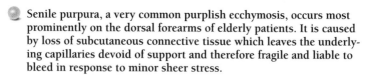 Senile purpura, a very common purplish ecchymosis, occurs most prominently on the dorsal forearms of elderly patients. It is caused by loss of subcutaneous connective tissue which leaves the underlying capillaries devoid of support and therefore fragile and liable to bleed in response to minor sheer stress.

No workup is required if the platelet count is normal and the patient is otherwise well.

In scurvy, the severe vitamin C deficiency results in poor connective tissue support of capillaries leading to a petechial and purpuric eruption.

In distinction to other causes of petechiae those associated with scurvy tend to be perifollicular and located on the dorsal, rather than the volar, aspect of the forearm. Large ecchymoses may occur in a saddle distribution involving the buttocks.

In acute meningococcemia, endotoxin and cytokines damage the endothelium and cause subcutaneous hemorrhage that begins as pink to red petechiae and coalesces to purpura over the course of minutes to hours.

DIC frequently contributes as well.

Endothelial damage is also the cause of petechiae and purpura in the viral hemorrhagic fevers such as Lassa fever and Ebola infections.

Again, DIC probably contributes.

OTHER CHANGES IN THE CELLULAR ELEMENTS OF THE BLOOD

Erythrocytosis

Polycythemia rubra vera, an increase in RBC mass, is a myeloproliferative disease; it needs to be distinguished from "stress polycythemia" in which the RBC mass is normal but the plasma volume is reduced, thereby increasing the concentration of Hgb and the hematocrit.

Determination of RBC mass with chromium 51-tagged RBCs and consideration of possible other causes will usually clarify the diagnosis. Chronic hypoxia, ectopic production of erythropoietin in paraneoplastic syndromes, and variant Hgbs with tight O_2 affinities are other causes of polycythemia.

Polycythemia vera is usually associated with other abnormalities like splenomegaly, increased uric acid, and physical findings such as ruddy complexion and tortuous and engorged retinal veins (sometimes leading to retinal vein thrombosis).

Hyperviscosity of the blood is noted with hematocrits above 50% and this predisposes to venous thrombosis of the hepatic and other veins.

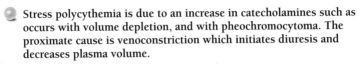 Stress polycythemia is due to an increase in catecholamines such as occurs with volume depletion, and with pheochromocytoma. The proximate cause is venoconstriction which initiates diuresis and decreases plasma volume.

The body has no direct means for assessing plasma volume; it uses the surrogate measure of pressure in the capacitance (central venous) portion of the circulation to infer volume status. Venoconstriction with increase in central venous pressure is read as a "full tank" when in fact it is just a smaller tank. Diuresis is thus the consequence of central venoconstriction.

Acute pancreatitis with exudation of large amounts of fluid in the inflamed abdominal space may be associated with impressive increases in the hematocrit.

Hematocrits of 60% and above may be seen in severe cases of pancreatitis, and indicates the need for aggressive volume repletion.

Thrombocytosis

Essential thrombocytosis is part of the spectrum of myeloproliferative diseases; it needs to be distinguished from various other nonmalignant causes of thrombocytosis.

Mild splenomegaly and leukocytosis are frequently associated with essential thrombocytosis. The platelet count exceeds 500,000. The complications are arterial thromboses and paradoxically, bleeding, when the platelet count exceeds one million; bleeding is due to alterations in vWF that occurs in essential thrombocytosis.

Nonmalignant thrombocytosis occurs with any inflammatory disease, post splenectomy, and with iron deficiency anemia.

The elevation is generally modest and thrombotic or bleeding complications do not occur.

Thrombocytosis in excess of 500,000 may be associated with "pseudohyperkalemia" due to release of potassium from platelets in clotted serum.

Measurement of potassium in plasma (as opposed to serum) establishes the true potassium level.

Neutropenias

Neutropenia, also known as granulocytopenia, although the latter technically refers to eosinophils and basophils as well as neutrophils, is defined as an absolute neutrophil count (ANC) below 1,500/μL. Agranulocytosis refers to an ANC of essentially zero.

Risk of bacterial or fungal infection increases significantly with ANC levels below 500. Viral infections are not impacted since these are defended by lymphocytic immune mechanisms.

Bone marrow evaluation distinguishes between failure of granulocyte development and peripheral destruction. In the presence of neutropenia of uncertain cause the threshold for obtaining a bone marrow aspirate and biopsy should be low.

Pharmaceuticals, a common cause of neutropenia, may affect neutrophil development in the marrow or cause peripheral destruction by immune mechanisms.

The list of agents, cancer chemotherapeutics aside, associated with neutropenia is huge. Agranulocytosis is associated with a smaller number of drugs including antithyroid agents, psychotropic agents, and chloramphenicol, the latter causing aplastic anemia as well and no longer in general use.

The manifestations of agranulocytosis include fever, sores in the mouth and on the gums, sore throat, and trouble swallowing. Patients on agents known to be associated with agranulocytosis need to be warned about the symptoms and instructed to discontinue the drug and call the physician should the above manifestations develop.

This is particularly true for the antithyroid drugs, especially propylthiouracil. These reactions are typically idiosyncratic and the warning is more important than repeated CBCs, although monitoring the latter is recommended as well.

Infections are common causes of neutropenia. Viral infections and severe bacterial infections are common offenders.

Neutropenia with bacterial sepsis has a poor prognosis.

Patients with pneumococcal pneumonia are noteworthy examples. Endotoxin from gram-negative organisms, particularly with gram-negative sepsis, is frequently associated with neutropenia. Typhoid fever is a good example where the manifestations of the illness, including neutropenia, reflect endotoxemia.

Hypersplenism is a prominent cause of pancytopenia affecting RBCs and platelets as well as neutrophils. Any disease associated with splenic enlargement may cause hypersplenism, although congestive splenomegaly from portal hypertension is the most common cause.

Deficiency of any of the formed elements of the blood may occur in hypersplenism, and in any combination.

Autoimmune neutropenia also occurs in association with several collagen vascular diseases, notably systemic lupus erythematosus and rheumatoid arthritis. Usually modest in degree, the neutropenia is analogous to acquired autoimmune hemolytic anemia and ITP.

In lupus patients under treatment the issue may arise as to the origin of a febrile episode. Is it a lupus flare or infection as a consequence of immunosuppression? In the absence of obvious sepsis, which may lower the WBC count, neutropenia favors a lupus flare.

Lymphopenia and Lymphocytosis

Immunosuppressive drugs such as azathioprine are commonly associated with lymphopenia.

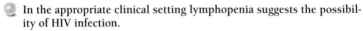 In the appropriate clinical setting lymphopenia suggests the possibility of HIV infection.

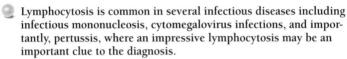 Lymphocytosis is common in several infectious diseases including infectious mononucleosis, cytomegalovirus infections, and importantly, pertussis, where an impressive lymphocytosis may be an important clue to the diagnosis.

Leukocytosis

Increases in circulating white blood cells (WBCs) may involve all leukocyte lineages. The particular white cell lines involved has important diagnostic implications.

 Leukemoid reaction refers to neutrophil counts above 25,000 to 50,000, along with the presence of immature neutrophil precursors on blood smear. The usual cause is severe infection.

Pneumococcal sepsis is a common cause in young patients and children.

 Leukemoid reactions can be distinguished from chronic myelocytic leukemia (CML) by leukocyte alkaline phosphatase, which is low in CML but elevated in leukemoid reactions.

CML may also be Philadelphia chromosome positive and has an increase in basophils.

 The term leukoerythroblastic reaction refers to nucleated red blood cells along with immature WBCs in the peripheral smear. It occurs with marrow infiltration (myelopthisis), myelofibrosis, or severe infection (sepsis, military TB).

A classic association is with military TB. Eleanor Roosevelt died of military TB with marrow involvement. The leukoerythroblastic reaction had led to the erroneous diagnosis of a hematologic malignancy.

 Eosinophilic leukocytosis occurs with allergic reactions, parasitic infestations (worms, not protozoans), and some collagen vascular diseases (Churg–Strauss syndrome).

The presence of eosinophils in the blood is a strong evidence against a pyogenic (bacterial) infection.

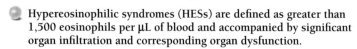

● Hypereosinophilic syndromes (HESs) are defined as greater than 1,500 eosinophils per μL of blood and accompanied by significant organ infiltration and corresponding organ dysfunction.

HES can be divided into primary, secondary, and idiopathic groups. The primary group is eosinophilia associated with a myeloproliferative disorder, usually a consequence of a chromosomal deletion resulting in constitutive activation of a tyrosine kinase. The abnormality is clonal and sometimes associated with blasts in the peripheral blood. In the secondary group an underlying disorder (parasitic infection, collagen vascular disease, malignancy) produces cytokines that stimulate the eosinophilia. If no cause can be identified the eosinophilia is termed "idiopathic."

● Pulmonary, cardiac, and gastrointestinal infiltration with eosinophils may be associated with significant morbidity and mortality.

Cardiac eosinophilic infiltration is particularly severe affecting both the coronary arteries and the myocardium with corresponding infarction, inflammation, and thrombus formation.

The lungs may be impacted by direct eosinophilic infiltration (chronic eosinophilic pneumonia) or with helminthic larval migration from the intestines to the venous blood and thence to the alveoli and up the respiratory tree to be swallowed and re-enter the gut. The latter, known as Löffler's syndrome, occurs with ascaris, hookworm, and *Strongyloides stercoralis* and may be asymptomatic or associated with cough dyspnea and, occasionally, hemoptysis.

● Strongyloides is unique in that the life cycle does not require another host, so autoinfection can occur.

Occasionally, particularly in immunosuppressed patients, a large parasite burden of eggs and larvae can result in strongyloides "hyperinfection," a serious complication with wide dissemination of the parasite. Strongyloides does occur in the southeastern part of the United States but is more common in immigrants from Southeast Asia.

● GI infiltration with eosinophils may result in abdominal pain, weight loss, vomiting, and diarrhea.

● Lymphocytic leukocytosis suggests infectious mononucleosis (EBV), pertussis, cytomegalovirus (CMV) infection, or chronic lymphocytic leukemia (CLL). Monocytosis suggests TB.

THROMBOTIC DISORDERS AND COAGULOPATHIES

Platelets provide the first line of defense in response to insults that cause bleeding. The subsequent development of a firm clot depends on normal blood coagulation. In addition to the well described inherited clotting factor deficiencies like classic hemophilia, several other acquired coagulopathies cause significant bleeding. At the other end of the spectrum a number of congenital or acquired diseases result in pathologic clotting and thromboembolic disease.

Prothrombotic Diatheses

Risk factors for the development of deep vein thrombosis (DVT) include stasis in the venous system, blood vessel damage, and hyper-coagulability of the blood (Virchow's triad). Older age independently increases the risk of DVT.

Thus, immobility, trauma, and factors that exert a prothrombotic effect, such as Factor V Leiden, antiphospholipid antibody syndrome, and estrogens all predispose to DVT and venous thromboembolism (VTE).

The most significant inherited hypercoagulable state is Factor V Leiden, a mutation that causes resistance of Factor V to inactivation by activated protein C and predisposes to venous thrombosis.

An autosomal dominant trait with variable expressivity Factor V Leiden occurs in the heterozygous state in about 5% of the United States population. The Factor V Leiden mutation is found in about one-quarter of patients presenting with DVT or VTE. Many individuals with the mutation do not experience DVTs. The much rarer homozygous state is associated with a considerably higher incidence of thrombosis.

The antiphospholipid syndrome (APS) is an autoimmune disease associated with both venous and arterial thromboses.

Pregnancy complications including fetal loss also occur as a clinical manifestation of APS.

The autoantibodies are directed against membrane phospholipids and their associated proteins.

The three antiphospholipid autoantibodies measured clinically are the lupus anticoagulant, the anticardiolipin antibody, and the anti–β2-glycoprotein antibody. (The "lupus anticoagulant" is a misnomer since it is associated with thromboses, not bleeding, and many patients with this antibody do not have lupus. It was called an anticoagulant since it falsely prolongs the PTT.) In addition to detecting these antibodies on two separate occasions the diagnosis of APS requires a clinical event (thrombosis or obstetric) since many normal people have antiphospholipid antibodies without evident disease.

The so-called primary APS occurs in the absence of other rheumatic diseases; secondary APS occurs in conjunction with other autoimmune diseases, most notably, lupus.

DVT is the most common venous thrombotic event and stroke the most common arterial event in patients having APS. Myocardial infarctions also occur.

Perhaps 10% to 15% of these thrombotic events occur in association with APS. It is not clear how these antibodies cause thromboses.

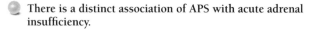 **There is a distinct association of APS with acute adrenal insufficiency.**

The adrenal lesion is infarction, either thrombotic or hemorrhagic. The latter may reflect adrenal vein thrombosis with consequent hemorrhagic infarction. Back pain and hypotension are early clues to the diagnosis, and indicate the need for a cosyntropin test.

Nephrotic syndrome causes a hypercoagulable state by the urinary loss of low molecular weight proteins that block coagulation, particularly, antithrombin III.

Increases in prothrombotic factors, including fibrinogen, also contribute. Perhaps one-quarter of patients with the nephrotic syndrome suffer thrombosis.

Renal vein thrombosis is particularly associated with the nephrotic syndrome since the deficiency of antithrombin III is greatest in blood draining the kidneys.

The procoagulant activity is therefore accentuated in the renal veins increasing the susceptibility to thromboses.

Coagulopathies

Circulating anticoagulants are autoantibodies that neutralize clotting factors and mimic congenital clotting factor deficiencies except for their initial occurrence in late adult life or after pregnancy. Antibody to Factor VIII is the most common.

The diagnosis of a circulating anticoagulant is made by a classic mixing study which tests the result of mixing a patient's blood with normal plasma. Unlike factor deficiencies the prolongation of the PTT in patients with a circulating anticoagulant is not corrected by a one-to-one dilution with normal plasma. The treatment is with immunosuppressants rather than factor replacement.

von Willebrand disease (vWD), a congenital deficiency of vWF, produces a mild bleeding diathesis by interfering with normal platelet adhesion at a site of injury.

The bleeding time is prolonged in vWD. Bruisability, heavy menstrual flow, and bleeding after surgical procedures are common manifestations. Factor VIII is modestly reduced in most cases as well. Replacement of vWF or the administration of DDAVP, which augments the release of vWF, constitutes treatment which may be required before surgical or dental procedures.

Rheumatology: Arthritis, Autoimmune and Collagen Vascular Diseases

ARTHRITIS

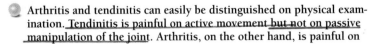 Arthritis and tendinitis can easily be distinguished on physical examination. Tendinitis is painful on active movement but not on passive manipulation of the joint. Arthritis, on the other hand, is painful on both active and passive movement.

It is important to distinguish tendinitis from actual joint involvement.

Osteoarthritis (Degenerative Joint Disease [DJD])

The most common rheumatologic disease is osteoarthritis, also called DJD. Although not an exciting disease entity it is a major cause of disability.

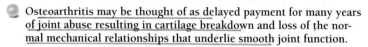 Osteoarthritis may be thought of as delayed payment for many years of joint abuse resulting in cartilage breakdown and loss of the normal mechanical relationships that underlie smooth joint function.

Knees and hips are common sites of involvement but no joint is immune. There is clearly a genetic component as well.

  Heberden's and Bouchard's nodes are common forms of osteoarthritis that present as deformed, nodular, bony swelling of the distal interphalangeal (DIP) and proximal interphalangeal (PIP) joints respectively.

Most common in elderly women, these nodes are not usually painful but may cause some loss of mobility.

  Baker's cyst may complicate osteoarthritis of the knee.

Almost any type of arthritis or injury to the knee may be associated with a Baker's cyst.

The cyst, which is located in the popliteal fossa and communicates with the joint space, may rupture resulting in painful inflammation of the calf. Swelling, pain, and tenderness with difficulty bearing weight are common consequences.

  A ruptured Baker's cyst may be erroneously confused with thrombophlebitis.

Ultrasound establishes the diagnosis of a ruptured Baker's cyst.

  Charcot joint, a particularly destructive variant of osteoarthritis, refers to extensive joint damage due to loss of proprioceptive innervation secondary to underlying neurologic disease.

Loss of proprioception subjects the joint to unusual stress which results, ultimately, in total joint destruction. The location of the damaged joint depends upon the underlying neurologic disease.

  The most common cause of Charcot joint at the ankle is diabetes; at the knee, syphilis (tabes dorsalis); at the shoulder or the elbow, syringomyelia; at the wrist Hansen's disease (leprosy, neuritic form).

Olecranon Bursitis

Olecranon bursitis, inflammation of the olecranon bursa accompanied by fluid accumulation, swelling, and often redness, is usually the result of acute or chronic traumatic injury.

🔹 Olecranon bursitis can be distinguished from arthritis of the elbow on physical examination: pronation and supination at the elbow joint cause pain if the elbow joint is involved; flexion and extension cause pain with both olecranon bursitis and elbow arthritis.

🔹 Olecranon bursitis may complicate rheumatoid arthritis (RA), often in relation to a subcutaneous nodule located over the bursa. Similarly, an overlying tophus in patients with gout may be associated with olecranon bursitis.

Olecranon bursitis may also be seen in alcoholics (elbows leaning on the bar!).

🔹 Infection may complicate olecranon bursitis if the skin splits; *Staphylococcus aureus* is the usual organism.

Rheumatoid Arthritis (RA)

RA is a systemic disease principally involving the synovia and the joints. The cause is unknown, but heredity, autoimmunity, infectious agents, and environmental (smoking) factors may play a role. The disease is more common in women especially in younger patients. HLA-DR4 is a common histocompatibility antigen in RA patients.

🔹 Rheumatoid factor (RF), an IgM antibody directed against gamma globulin, is useful diagnostically although the sensitivity and specificity depend on the prior probability of the disease.

RF has been a biomarker for RA for over half a century. Recently, anticyclic citrullinated antibodies (anti-CCP) have been utilized as a diagnostic test. In patients with inflammatory arthritis the sensitivity of RF is about 70% and the specificity about 85%. The higher the titer the greater is the specificity of RF for RA. Anti-CCP antibodies appear to have a similar sensitivity and slightly greater specificity.

🔹 RF is also positive in other collagen vascular diseases and in some chronic infectious diseases.

Thus, Sjögren's syndrome, Lupus, and subacute bacterial endocarditis are not infrequently RF positive.

🔹 Approximately 50% of patients with RA are RF negative at the time of presentation.

RF positivity subsequently develops in many patients as the disease progresses. The role of RF in the pathogenesis of RA, if any, is unknown.

🔹 High-titer RF is associated with long-standing disease, aggressive joint destruction, subcutaneous nodules, vasculitis, and other extra-articular manifestations.

🔹 The small joints of the hands, wrists, feet, and ankles are the most common sites of involvement in RA, although involvement of larger joints (knees, hips, elbows, and spine) also occurs.

🔵 **At the ankle the subtalar joints are most prominently involved affecting inversion and eversion more than flexion and extension.**

Characteristic deformities of the hands (ulna deviation, swan neck deformities), bilateral wrist involvement, and bony erosions on x-ray help establish the diagnosis.

🔵 **Morning stiffness, although not specific for RA, is characteristic.**

The stiffness is not fleeting; it lasts at least 1 hour.

🔵 **Although RA is most common in middle-aged women, extra-articular manifestations are more common in older men.**

🔵 **Extra-articular manifestations are associated with severe articular disease, subcutaneous nodules, and high-titer rheumatoid factor (Table 3-1).**

Subcutaneous nodules occur most frequently on extensor surfaces around the hands and elbow, but histologically, similar rheumatoid nodules may occur in viscera as well, including the heart and lungs.

🔵 **Cardiac rheumatoid nodules, if strategically located around the conducting system, may cause heart block. Rheumatoid nodules may also, uncommonly, occur in the lung.**

🔵 **Rheumatoid pleural effusion is exudative and characterized by an extremely low glucose level, a low complement level, and a low pH.**

RF in the pleural fluid may be positive as well. The pH may be very low and may require repeated thoracentesis to avoid the development of a fibrothorax.

🔵 **Bi-basilar pulmonary fibrosis is the most common form of pulmonary involvement in RA.**

It predisposes to pneumonia which may require a long course of treatment. This is particularly true in the face of immunosuppressive treatment or when neutropenia is present (Felty's syndrome).

TABLE 3.1 Extra-articular Manifestations of RA

High-titer Rheumatoid Factor

• Subcutaneous nodules	• Bibasilar pulmonary fibrosis
• Visceral rheumatoid nodules	• Mononeuritis multiplex
• Rheumatoid vasculitis	• Felty's syndrome
▫ Digital arteries	▫ Splenomegaly
▫ Coronaries	▫ Neutropenia
• Rheumatoid pleural effusion	
▫ Exudative	
▫ Low complement	
▫ Low pH	

- Rheumatoid vasculitis occurs in the course of aggressive disease with high-titer rheumatoid factor, and is often associated with characteristic linear ulcerations around the digital arteries of the terminal phalanges of the hands.

- Rheumatoid vasculitis of the coronary arteries may cause myocardial ischemia and infarction, and vasculitis of the vasa vasorum of major motor nerves may cause nerve infarction and the corresponding syndrome of mononeuritis multiplex.

Rheumatoid vasculitis involving the kidneys is vanishingly rare.

- Felty's syndrome, a triad including RA, splenomegaly, and neutropenia, occurs most commonly in long-standing RA with high-titer rheumatoid factor and other extra-articular manifestations.

Antineutrophil antibodies and splenic sequestration explain the neutropenia.

- The possibility of septic arthritis masquerading as an RA flare should be considered, particularly in febrile patients with acute joint symptoms.

Since RA patients are often on an immunosuppressive regimen, joint infections that mimic a flare in the underlying disease may occur. These infections are usually caused by *S. aureus,* are associated with *S. aureus* bacteremia, and usually involve large joints such as hip or knee.

- Consider palindromic rheumatism in the differential diagnosis of RA in patients who have recurrent bouts of acute arthritis, are RF negative, and have no joint deformities.

Palindromic rheumatism is an acute inflammatory arthritis that is evanescent, recurs at variable intervals, and does not result in chronic joint deformity. The cause is unknown.

Adult Still's Disease (Juvenile Rheumatoid Arthritis)

- Previously known as juvenile rheumatoid arthritis (JRA), Adult Still's disease is a prominent cause of undiagnosed febrile illness in young adults.

- Diagnosis is purely clinical and supported by a distinctive fever pattern of two spikes per day and by the recognition of an evanescent pale erythematous maculopapular eruption, most commonly noted on the trunk, particularly in areas subject to pressure, such as the back.

Other clues to the diagnosis include pharyngitis early in the course, arthralgias (and occasionally, arthritis), and very high levels of inflammatory indices including, importantly, very high ferritin levels. The latter are usually elevated out of proportion to other indices of inflammation. RF is negative.

Psoriatic Arthritis

- An asymmetric RF-negative, spondyloarthropathy, psoriatic arthritis affects principally the distal phalangeal joints and is associated with pitting of the finger nails and onycholysis.

Although it is associated with psoriasis, in a small minority of patients, the joint disease may antedate the skin disease. It is commonly associated with HLA-B27 tissue type and sacroiliitis is a common accompaniment.

Reactive Arthritis

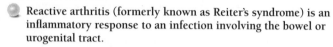 Reactive arthritis (formerly known as Reiter's syndrome) is an inflammatory response to an infection involving the bowel or urogenital tract.

The inciting infections include those caused by *Chlamydia, Campylobacter, Shigella, Yersinia,* and *Salmonella* species.

 The arthritis, which usually favors the large joints of the lower extremities, is mono- or oligoarticular and asymmetric; it is variable in severity, and occurs principally, but not exclusively, in patients positive for HLA-B27.

The sacroiliac joints and the spine may be involved. The infection frequently precedes the arthritis by 1 to several weeks. Reactive arthritis following genitourinary infections has a marked male predominance (10 to 1 or greater), but the syndrome following enteric infections affects women equally.

 In addition to arthritis, the skin, the eyes, and the mucous membranes may be involved.

The triad of urethritis, arthritis, and conjunctivitis was previously known as Reiter's syndrome.

 The characteristic skin lesions often associated with Reiter's syndrome go by the colorful name keratoderma blenorrhagica; they are papulosquamous lesions with a serpiginous border classically located on the soles and palms.

The eye inflammation involves the anterior chamber and may vary between mild conjunctivitis and severe anterior uveitis.

 Shallow erosions on the penis are known as circinate balanitis.

In circumcised men lesions on the shaft of the penis resemble the keratoderma described above.

Crystal Deposition Arthridities: Uric Acid and Calcium Pyrophosphate

 Gout is a severe monoarticular arthritis, characteristically involving the metatarsophalangeal joint of the big toe (podagra).

The inflammation is so intense that even the bed sheets on the affected joint cannot be tolerated. The knee, the dorsum of the foot, the ankle joint (mortise and tenon portion affecting flexion and extension) and the instep are sites of involvement as well.

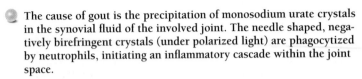 **The cause of gout is the precipitation of monosodium urate crystals in the synovial fluid of the involved joint. The needle shaped, negatively birefringent crystals (under polarized light) are phagocytized by neutrophils, initiating an inflammatory cascade within the joint space.**

Hyperuricemia is the underlying cause, but during an acute attack the serum uric acid level need not be elevated. Demonstration of phagocytized crystals in the joint fluid secures the diagnosis.

Acute gouty attacks are frequently precipitated by unrelated hospitalization, surgery, and generous alcohol intake.

It is not unusual for the first attack to occur when the patient wakes from anesthesia after surgery for an unrelated problem.

Ethanol increases plasma lactate which inhibits the tubular excretion of urate, a change that may precipitate an acute attack of gout.

The initiation of uricosuric therapy, or the inhibition of urate synthesis with allopurinol, mobilizes urate from tissue stores in tophi and may induce an acute attack. Prophylactic administration of colchicine or nonsteroidal anti-inflammatory agents is indicated when treatment to lower uric acid levels is initiated.

Tophi, the precipitation of monosodium urate in soft tissues, develop after years of hyperuricemia; they occur most commonly adjacent to joints and in the skin of the ear lobe over the auricular cartilage.

Chronic tophaceous gout refers to polyarticular arthritis that occurs in relation to tophaceous deposits around joints which may result in destructive changes. In distinction to acute gout joint involvement with tophi may cause a chronic arthritis in multiple joints reminiscent of osteoarthritis.

Gout is a disease of men and to a lesser extent of postmenopausal women. It is associated with obesity, hypertension, and diabetes mellitus.

High-serum uric acid is a risk factor for cardiovascular disease, for reasons that remain obscure.

Pseudogout is an acute arthritis usually involving the knee or wrist caused by the precipitation of calcium pyrophosphate dihydrate in the synovial space.

It is a disease of the elderly, and men and women are equally affected. There is an association with hyperparathyroidism, hemochromatosis, and osteoarthritis. Decreased levels of phosphatases in the articular cartilage with aging may contribute.

Acute inflammation is caused by the phagocytosis of rhomboid-shaped positively birefringent calcium pyrophosphate crystals (under polarized light).

The disease is frequently chronic and may involve multiple joints. Treatment of the acute attack is similar to that of gout.

Chondrocalcinosis, a linear deposition of calcium in the articular cartilage of the involved joint, helps confirm the diagnosis of pseudogout; chondrocalcinosis, however, is common in the elderly, frequently asymptomatic, and often occurs without pseudogout.

ANCA-ASSOCIATED VASCULITIDES

Wegener's granulomatosis (granulomatosis with polyangiitis [GPA]), microscopic polyangiitis (MPA), and Churg–Strauss syndrome (CSS) are the major vasculitides associated with positive antineutrophil cytoplasmic antibodies (Table 3-2).

Antineutrophil cytoplasmic antibodies (ANCAs), IgG autoantibodies directed against proteinase 3 (c-ANCA, cytoplasmic immunostaining), or myeloperoxidase (p-ANCA, perinuclear immunostaining), are present in the blood of many patients with systemic vasculitis. They are useful diagnostically even if their specific role in the pathogenesis of vasculitis is uncertain.

c-ANCA is highly associated with Wegener's granulomatosis; p-ANCA is less specific but associated more with MPA; the CSS may be associated with either.

TABLE 3.2 ANCA-associated Vasculitides

Disease	Distinguishing Features
Wegener's granulomatosis (granulomatosis with polyangiitis [GPA])	C-ANCA positive, necrotizing granulomas, history of nasal polyps, oral ulcerations, episcleritis, cavitary lung lesions, mononeuritis multiplex
Microscopic polyangiitis (MPA)	P-ANCA or C-ANCA positive, absent granulomas, interstitial pulmonary fibrosis, mononeuritis multiplex
Churg–Strauss syndrome (CSS) also known as eosinophilic granulomatosis with polyangiitis (EGPA)	P-ANCA positive in 50%, eosinophilia, asthma, rhinitis, cardiac involvement, mononeuritis multiplex

Wegener's Granulomatosis (Granulomatosis with Polyangiitis [GPA])

Wegener's granulomatosis, a necrotizing granulomatous polyangiitis of the small- and midsized vessels, is characterized by involvement of the upper airway, the lungs, and the kidneys. Small- to medium-sized vessels are involved.

- Distinctive features that suggest the diagnosis of Wegener's granulomatosis are sinusitis, nasal polyps, oral ulcerations, ocular lesions (prominently, episcleritis), ear involvement (otitis media), glomerulonephritis, mononeuritis multiplex, and the presence of necrotizing granulomas on biopsy.

- A history of nasal polyps and sinusitis are important clues to the diagnosis of Wegener's granulomatosis (GPA).

- Pulmonary lesions in Wegener's granulomatosis are highly variable but cavitary nodules are especially characteristic.

The glomerulonephritis is "pauci-immune" in that it does not involve immune complex deposition. Biopsies of affected tissues reveal granulomas, necrosis, and vasculitis. Cytoplasmic antineutrophil antibodies to proteinase 3 (c-ANCA) are usually positive and very helpful diagnostically.

This disease was rapidly fatal before the important discovery that Cytoxan was highly efficacious in producing long-term remissions.

Microscopic Polyangiitis (MPA)

- MPA resembles Wegener's granulomatosis in many respects; the absence of granulomas in MPA, however, distinguishes the two entities on histologic grounds.

Other points of distinction include the lung involvement.

- In MPA, interstitial fibrosis is the usual lesion rather than the characteristic cavitary nodules of Wegener's granulomatosis.

As compared with Wegener's granulomatosis, MPA has a higher incidence of mononeuritis multiplex, and is less likely to relapse after successful treatment.

Churg–Strauss Syndrome (CSS)

- CSS, also known as eosinophilic granulomatosis with polyangiitis (EGPA), is characterized by asthma, eosinophilia, and tissue infiltration with eosinophils.

- Asthma and rhinitis are usually the first manifestation of CSS, followed by eosinophilia and vasculitis.

ANCA positivity is present in only one-half of the patients. Pulmonary involvement consists of fleeting infiltrates; there is a high incidence of mononeuritis multiplex, and renal involvement is less severe than in Wegener's granulomatosis or MPA.

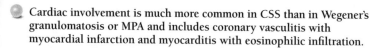

Cardiac involvement is much more common in CSS than in Wegener's granulomatosis or MPA and includes coronary vasculitis with myocardial infarction and myocarditis with eosinophilic infiltration.

Involvement of the heart is a major cause of death in patients with severe CSS.

Vasculitis of the vasa nervorum leads to infarction of major motor nerves (including cranial nerves); the resulting clinical syndrome, known as mononeuritis multiplex, is very common in CSS and MPA, and less so in Wegener's granulomatosis.

Drug-induced ANCA–Associated Vasculitis (AAV)

Drug-induced vasculitis associated with p-ANCA resembles MPA.

Glomerulonephritis and alveolar hemorrhage from pulmonary capillary inflammation are the most serious manifestations of drug-induced AAV.

Many drugs have been implicated in AAV, but hydralazine is a major offender along with propylthiouracil, other antithyroid drugs, allopurinol, and anti–TNF-α agents.

NON-ANCA–ASSOCIATED VASCULITIDES

Behcet's Syndrome

A small-vessel vasculitis, Behcet's syndrome is characterized by mucosal ulcerations (mouth and genital), arthritis, uveitis, and occasionally CNS involvement (chronic meningoencephalitis, dural vein thrombosis).

Behcet's syndrome is rare in the United States and Western Europe, but common in the Middle East, particularly Turkey.

Eye involvement may be severe and cause blindness. Other manifestations include ulcerations in the GI tract, hemoptysis, pleuritis, and aneursyms of the pulmonary artery.

In the United States most suspected cases of Behcet's disease turn out to be Crohn's disease.

Some patients with self-inflected wounds (factitious disease) may also be suspected of Behcet's disease.

Cryoglobulinemia

Cryoglobulinemia results from the reversible precipitation of immunoglobulin complexes (cryoglobulins) at lower than normal body temperatures. The immunoglobulin is either a monoclonal paraprotein from malignant plasma cells or a polyclonal aggregation of IgG and IgM directed at various antigens. Hepatitis C antigens are most commonly involved.

Cryoglobulins are distinct from cold agglutinins which are autoantibodies directed at RBC membranes that precipitate at reduced temperature.

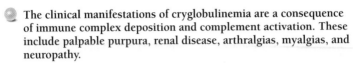 The clinical manifestations of cryglobulinemia are a consequence of immune complex deposition and complement activation. These include palpable purpura, renal disease, arthralgias, myalgias, and neuropathy.

Giant Cell Arteritis (GCA)

Temporal arteritis is a granulomatous GCA involving the extracranial branches of the aorta and, rarely, the aorta itself.

- Headache, fever, and a very high sedimentation rate are usually present.
- Jaw claudication during mastication (masseter muscle ischemia) is a specific symptom.
- The feared complication is blindness from involvement of the ophthalmic circulation.

Visual symptoms with headache should be considered a medical emergency. Temporal artery biopsy frequently (but not always) secures the diagnosis of GCA. High-dose steroid (60-mg prednisone per day) is effective treatment. The dose is tapered down following symptoms and ESR. Remission usually occurs after 1 or 2 years.

- The spectrum of GCA includes polymyalgia rheumatica (PMR), characterized by stiffness and pain in the axial skeleton (hip and shoulder girdle), worse in the morning.
- Alkaline phosphatase elevation is not uncommon in PMR.
- The diagnosis of PMR is based on the clinical findings rather than biopsy.

Prompt symptomatic relief in response to corticosteroids is typical. Low doses may be used in PMR (20-mg prednisone per day) in distinction to the cranial arteritis form of the disease where high initial doses are appropriate. The goal is symptomatic relief and reduction (if not normalization) of the ESR.

COLLAGEN VASCULAR DISEASES

Scleroderma (Systemic Sclerosis)

Literally hardened or thickened skin, scleroderma is a fibrosing disease with deposition of collagen in the skin and other organs. The cause is unknown, but autoimmunity, genetics, and environmental factors are seemingly involved.

- CREST syndrome represents a limited form of scleroderma with slow progression.

Calcinosis cutis, Raynaud's syndrome, Esophageal dysmotility, Sclerodactyly, and Telangiectasias occur as a constellation and herald a long course with a better prognosis than the diffuse form of the disease. Pulmonary hypertension occurs in a minority of cases of the CREST syndrome.

- **Calcinosis cutis consists of powdery or speculated calcium crystals that break through the skin, usually at the finger tips.**

- **Sclerodactyly is a hallmark of scleroderma and should be a clue to the diagnosis early in the disease presentation; inability to make a fist is an early physical finding.**

Tightening of the skin of the hands and atrophy of the underlying digital muscles results in a claw-like appearance of the hands.

- **Raynaud's phenomenon (pain and whitening of the fingers on exposure to cold) is often the first manifestation of scleroderma.**

The diagnosis of scleroderma is frequently made by recognition of early sclerodactyly in a patient with Raynaud's syndrome. Many patients, of course, have Raynaud's syndrome without evidence of systematic disease.

Beta-blockers accentuate peripheral vasoconstriction and are contraindicated in Raynaud's disease.

- **Telangiectasias, dilated capillary loops, are located principally at the base of the nail beds; these may be quite prominent, but are not specific for scleroderma.**

Similar telangiectasias are found in other collagen vascular diseases as well.

- **Involvement of the GI tract in systemic sclerosis may be associated with serious motility problems. Dysphagia from esophageal involvement and malabsorption from bacterial overgrowth in the small intestine are common consequences of GI involvement in scleroderma.**

Malabsorption is due to bacterial deconjugation of bile acid salts with impaired micelle formation. The bacteria may also utilize nutrients such as vitamin B_{12}.

- **Skin involvement on the trunk and proximal extremities in patients with scleroderma herald a rapid course with visceral involvement and early demise.**

- **Scleroderma renal crisis is a serious development and occurs in the context of diffuse disease.**

Involvement of the renal vasculature with onion skin-like changes and fibrinoid necrosis reminiscent of malignant hypertension herald the rapid decline in renal function that occurs with the systemic form of the disease, the so-called scleroderma renal crisis. Treatment with an angiotensin converting enzyme (ACE) inhibitor is effective at improving renal function and treating hypertension in scleroderma patients.

- **Corticosteroids are contraindicated in scleroderma and they increase the risk of renal crisis.**

Polyarteritis Nodosa (PAN)

- A necrotizing vasculitis of the medium-sized arteries, PAN has no distinctive serologic markers.

- Angiographic demonstration of a characteristic aneurysmal beading of the vessels supplying the gut and kidneys helps secure the diagnosis.

In addition to systemic manifestations such as fever and weight loss the clinical features of PAN reflect the organs involved in the vasculitic process. Hemorrhage, hypertension, and renal insufficiency are commonly found. Involvement of the skin and peripheral nerves (mononeuritis multiplex) is also common.

- A significant number of cases of PAN, albeit a minority, occur in association with hepatitis B (HBV) infection.

Immune complex deposition in vessel walls may initiate the vasculitis in these cases.

Treatment is with corticosteroids (and cyclophosphamide in refractory cases), although steroids may exacerbate the hypertension that often accompanies PAN. In patients with the HBV-associated disease antiviral agents are given as well.

Polymyositis

- Weakness is the cardinal manifestation of polymyositis.

- The proximal musculature is affected the most. Weakness of the neck flexors is particularly prominent. Muscle tenderness occurs in a minority of patients.

- The notion that muscle tenderness is common in polymyositis is a *faux pearl*.

Creative kinase (CK) levels are usually elevated but do not correlate with the extent of the disease. Polymyositis may be associated with other collagen vascular diseases, especially scleroderma.

- The risk of malignancy in association with polymyositis is only slightly increased if at all.

Dermatomyositis (DM)

DM is a distinct disease from polymyositis with different muscle pathology and different disease associations.

- The characteristic skin lesions make the diagnosis of DM: violaceous rash about the eyes (so-called heliotrope), erythematous eruption in a v-shape on the upper chest, erythema over the shoulders posteriorly (shawl sign), and scaly red lesions over the knuckles (Gottron's papules).

CK levels in DM do not correlate with weakness or muscle involvement; in some cases, CK may be normal.

Telangiectasias of the nail beds are also common, but characteristic of other collagen vascular diseases as well.

🔵 **The incidence of malignancy in adults with DM is increased.**

About 15% of adult patients will have a malignancy diagnosed 1 to 2 years before or after the diagnosis of DM is established. Adenocarcinomas of the ovaries, stomach, breast, and colon are the most common cancers. These can usually be diagnosed on routine clinical evaluation with age-appropriate screening.

Systemic Lupus Erythematosus (SLE)

A systemic disease with protean manifestations and a variable, relapsing course, SLE affects many organ systems. Young women are predominantly affected.

🔵 **The usual manifestations of SLE are well known and include serositis, arthralgias, polyarthritis, rash, mucosal ulcerations, nephritis and nephrotic syndrome, sun sensitivity, leukopenia, autoimmune hemolytic anemia, and thrombocytopenia, among others.**

Serologic testing in the appropriate clinical context is the way that the diagnosis is established.

🔵 **The antinuclear antibody (ANA) is nonspecific but almost invariably positive in SLE. Very high-titer ANA has greater specificity. The double stranded DNA (dsDNA) is highly specific for SLE but lacks sensitivity; negative dsDNA by no means rules out the diagnosis.**

🔵 **Low complement levels are usual in the presence of active disease.**

A significant problem in SLE patients is separating a lupus flare from intercurrent infections or side effects of medications.

🔵 **Neuropsychiatric symptoms are relatively common in patients with SLE including seizures, headache, change in affect, poor cognition, confusion, and obtundation. These are frequently accompanied by fever and the clinical problem is to distinguish lupus cerebritis from CNS infection or steroid psychosis.**

Before these symptoms can be attributed to SLE cerebritis infectious causes have to be ruled out along with attendant metabolic abnormalities that may affect the CNS in lupus patients. Herpes encephalitis and toxoplasmosis are two treatable diseases that need to be excluded. Characteristic MRI findings may be helpful in distinguishing these since lupus cerebritis does not produce a distinctive MRI picture. Steroid psychosis usually occurs with high doses and manifests early in the course of treatment.

🔵 **The glomerulonephritis associated with SLE is due to immune complex deposition.**

The complex formed by autoantibodies directed to dsDNA appears to play a prominent role in the pathogenesis of lupus nephritis. The mesangium, subepithelium, subendothelium, or the glomerular basement membrane may be involved.

 Pulmonary involvement in SLE is common; pleuritis with or without effusion is the usual manifestation. Lupus pneumonitis or diffuse alveolar hemorrhage are uncommon but grave complications of SLE.

The pleural effusion has low complement levels. Pericarditis is not uncommon as well. Alveolar hemorrhage tends to be diffuse, with or without hemoptysis; an elevated diffusing capacity of the lungs for carbon monoxide (DLCO) and bronchoalveolar lavage may help confirm the diagnosis.

 Sun exposure is a well-known aggravating factor in SLE and should be avoided. Less well-known, but also important, is the need to avoid sulfa drugs which may also induce flares in the disease perhaps by sensitizing to sunlight.

Drug-induced Lupus

ANA is positive in drug-induced lupus; anti-dsDNA is usually but not always negative. Antihistone antibodies are usually positive in the drug-induced syndrome.

 Procainamide and hydralazine are the most common causes of drug-induced lupus. Arthralgias and myalgias, fever, and weight loss are the most common complaints. Serositis is more common with procainamide; rash with hydralazine.

As compared with SLE, drug-induced lupus occurs later in life, rarely involves the kidneys, the blood, or the CNS, and complement levels are normal. Slow acetylators are much more likely to develop drug-induced lupus from hydralazine or procainamide. The manifestations subside when the offending agent is withdrawn.

AMYLOIDOSIS

Amyloidosis, an accumulation of an abnormal fibrillar protein in different tissues, has historically been classified as primary and secondary (Table 3-3). A better understanding of the structure of amyloid has led to a different classification based on the structural characteristics and the origin of the abnormal protein. Overproduction and faulty processing (misfolding) of a normal protein resulting in the formation of the insoluble fibrillar amyloid protein is the usual cause.

The clinical picture presented by amyloidosis depends upon the location of the abnormal insoluble protein which infiltrates tissues and disrupts normal organ function. Amyloid in tissue samples stains with Congo red dye. Tissue

TABLE 3.3 Systemic Amyloidosis

Primary amyloidosis (AL) Plasma cell dyscrasia with overproduction of light chains that aggregate into insoluble fibrils	**Cardiac involvement** • Infiltrative restrictive cardiomyopathy with CHF **GI tract** • Motility disturbance with malabsorption from bacterial overgrowth **Kidneys** • Glomerular infiltration with nephrotic syndrome
Secondary amyloidosis (AA) The abnormal protein is an acute phase reactant (serum amyloid A) produced in chronic inflammatory states	**GI tract, liver, spleen, and kidneys most frequently involved** Large firm liver and spleen on examination
Systemic senile amyloidosis (SSA, ATTR) The abnormal protein is a misfolded transthyretin (TTR)	**Infiltrative restrictive cardiomyopathy in older men**
Familial amyloidosis (ATTR) Mutant ATTR	**Onset in young adults; peripheral nervous system involvement**

infiltration may occur from locally produced amyloid or from amyloid derived from the circulation.

Primary Amyloidosis (AL)

 AL is the consequence of a plasma cell dyscrasia with the overproduction of clonal light chains and is referred to as AL. The heart, the kidneys, and the GI tract are prominent cites of involvement.

Abnormal folding of the light chains in AL results in aggregation and the formation of insoluble protein fibrils that precipitate in tissues. Diagnosis is confirmed by demonstration of plasma cell dyscrasia and deposition of light chains in tissues.

 The corresponding AL manifestations are predictable and include infiltrative cardiomyopathy with heart failure; gut motility disturbances with constipation, diarrhea, or malabsorption; and nephrotic syndrome from renal glomerular infiltration. The tongue may also be infiltrated.

AL is in the differential diagnosis of macroglossia.

Secondary Amyloidosis (AA)

Secondary (reactive) amyloidosis occurs as a complication of long-standing inflammatory diseases such as RA and Crohn's disease. The amyloid protein deposition in this form of the disease is the acute-phase reactant serum amyloid A (SAA) and the designation is thus AA.

SAA, synthesized in the liver, is stimulated by a variety of proinflammatory cytokines.

Organ infiltration in AA involves the gut, the liver, the spleen, and the kidneys.

Familial Mediterranean fever (FMF) is a periodic inflammatory poly-serositis, due to a specific genetic abnormality. AA is an invariable complication of FMF.

Abdominal pain is a very common symptom of FMF; many patients will have had exploratory laparotomies for suspected acute appendicitis, and amyloid can frequently be detected in tissues removed at operation.

The inflammation in FMF responds to colchicine. Nephrotic syndrome from renal AA is a common complication.

Localized forms of amyloidosis exist as well; in medullary carcinoma of the thyroid, for example, the hormone calcitonin, produced by the tumor, is the responsible protein.

The amyloid in this case is limited to the thyroid.

Familial (ATTR) and Senile Amyloidosis (ATTRw)

The abnormal protein in senile amyloidosis is transthyretin (TTR), a prealbumin that carries thyroid hormones in the blood, and the corresponding amyloid is ATTR. This form of amyloid is the offending agent in familial and senile amyloidosis. In familial amyloidosis there is a mutation in the gene encoding ATTR resulting in a structurally abnormal protein; in senile amyloidosis it appears that the unmutated ATTR protein (wild type, ATTRw) becomes structurally unstable and abnormally folded.

Familial amyloidosis is a rare hereditable disease that usually manifests itself in early adulthood; the nervous system is the principle site of involvement, but the blood vessels and heart and the kidneys may be affected as well.

The principle clinical findings are polyneuropathy that affects the sensory, motor, and autonomic nervous systems. The inheritance is autosomal dominant.

Senile systemic amyloidosis (SSA) is a disease of older men principally affecting the heart.

The clinical features are those of a restrictive cardiomyopathy. As compared with AL amyloidosis the prognosis is better, macroglossia is absent, but an association with carpal tunnel syndrome is sometimes noted.

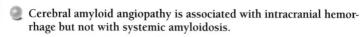 Cerebral amyloid angiopathy is associated with intracranial hemor-
rhage but not with systemic amyloidosis.

Amyloid deposition in the cerebral vessels is the cause.

IgG4-RELATED DISEASE

IgG4, a minor subclass of IgG, is produced under the influence of cytokines
derived from type 2 helper T cells. Its role in normal physiology remains
obscure. It has recently been identified as a cause of a number of poorly understood fibrosing diseases.

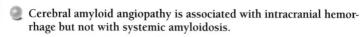 Retroperitoneal fibrosis, mediastinal fibrosis, pseudotumor of the
orbit, and autoimmune pancreatitis are some of the entities that fall
into the classification of IgG4-related disease.

Although serum IgG4 levels are frequently elevated the diagnosis requires his-
topathologic demonstration of characteristic fibrosis and tumefaction and a
dense plasmalymphocytic infiltrate that stains positive for IgG4.

PAGET'S DISEASE OF BONE

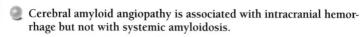 An elevated alkaline phosphatase level on multiphasic screening
tests is frequently the presenting manifestation.

A disorder of bone remodeling in aged individuals, the elevated alkaline
phosphatase level (bone isoform) reflects osteoblastic activity, although the
initial abnormality appears to be osteoclast regulation. The long bones of
the legs, the skull, and the pelvis are most frequently involved. Although the
bones appear sclerotic on x-ray pagetic bone is weak and subject to fracture.

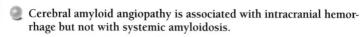 The clinical manifestations include nerve entrapment (deafness and
spinal stenosis), and rarely, hypercalcemia, in the presence of pro-
longed immobilization.

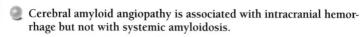 Increasing hat size in an elderly adult suggests the diagnosis.

Osteosarcoma is a rare complication.

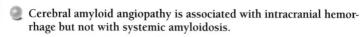 The radiologic appearance, particularly in the pelvis, is reminiscent
of metastatic prostate cancer.

Prostate cancer is easily distinguished by prostate-specific antigen (PSA) and
acid phosphatase levels.

SEVERE DRUG REACTIONS

The most common drug reaction is a blanching, erythematous, morbilliform,
maculopapular eruption that usually begins on the trunk. Fever is also a

common manifestation of drug allergy and may occur with or without a rash. Some less common drug reactions are life threatening: the DRESS syndrome and anaphylaxis are not common but are very serious.

THE DRESS SYNDROME (DRUG REACTION, RASH, EOSINOPHILIA, SYSTEMIC SYMPTOMS)

- The defining characteristics of severe drug-induced hypersensitivity reactions include a temporal relationship to an offending agent that begins after a latent period of 2 to 3 weeks, fever, rash, lymphadenopathy, eosinophilia, and evidence of internal organ involvement. Atypical lymphocytes, lymphopenia, or lymphocytosis may be prominent as well.

The cause is a specific immune reaction to the offending drug, although reactivation of latent herpes virus infection may also play a role.

- The common drugs causing severe hypersensitivity reactions include anticonvulsants (phenytoin, carbamazepine, and phenobarbital), allopurinol, sulfonamides, and antibiotics (minocycline, vancomycin, and beta-lactams).

The reaction may take weeks or even months to subside after the offending agent has been discontinued.

- Systemic involvement most commonly includes hepatitis, pneumonitis, and interstitial nephritis.

Corticosteroids are usually employed for systemic manifestation.

Anaphylactic Reactions

- Anaphylaxis is an acute, frequently life-threatening, IgE-mediated hypersensitivity reaction that results from mast cell degranulation with inflammatory mediator release.

Food allergies are common causes in children. In adults, drug reactions and venom from insect stings are the most common causes.

- Anaphylactoid reaction refers to non-IgE–mediated mast cell degranulation which is clinically indistinguishable from anaphylaxis.

Radiographic contrast media is the most common offender, but vancomycin and opioids may also cause anaphylactoid reactions.

- The clinical manifestations of anaphylaxis include flushing, hives and angioedema; wheezing and stridor; hypotension and shock.

- The most commonly associated drugs include penicillin and other beta-lactam antibiotics and NSAIDs.

● Every system review enquiry for drug allergy should include the question "Have you ever had penicillin? Did you have a reaction?" and the answers recorded in the record.

● Epinephrine is the specific antidote for anaphylaxis. Immediate intramuscular injection (anterior lateral thigh) is frequently lifesaving.

In the presence of shock intravenous epinephrine may be required. Patients with a history of anaphylactic reactions should carry an EpiPen on their person. The H-1 blocker diphenhydramine may be administered as well, but epinephrine is the critical treatment.

The Heart and Circulation

CHAPTER 4

CONGESTIVE HEART FAILURE (CHF)

The Pathophysiology of Heart Failure

CHF has increased in frequency with the aging of the population and now constitutes a major cause of cardiovascular morbidity and mortality. Hypertension is the major risk factor for CHF.

 The underlying hemodynamic abnormality in heart failure is an increase in ventricular end diastolic pressure.

Many descriptors have been applied to the failing heart based on the presumed underlying physiology: left heart failure, right heart failure, forward failure, congestive failure, diastolic dysfunction (heart failure with preserved ejection fraction), systolic failure (heart failure with diminished ejection fraction), to name a few. The common denominator is a rise in end diastolic pressure. This rise in pressure is transmitted backward to the atria and feeding veins resulting in pulmonary or systemic congestion with attendant dyspnea and edema.

 CHF is associated with increased sympathetic nervous system (SNS) activity. Tachycardia and enhanced cardiac contractility increase cardiac output.

The SNS stimulation is advantageous up to a point; if overly intense the resulting tachycardia and force of contraction may become disadvantageous by increasing the myocardial need for oxygen; hence the rationale for β-blockers. Antagonizing the inotropic effect of the SNS, however, may worsen failure, necessitating care in the use of β-blockers in patients with CHF.

A sign of CHF, hepatojugular reflux, is a manifestation of increased SNS tone.

When pressure is exerted on a congested liver, blood is forced into the superior vena cava; this increased volume in the capacitance veins results in a rise in venous pressure and an upward distention of the column of blood in the jugular veins. The increase in SNS activity increases the venous tone, so the jugular veins cannot accommodate the influx of blood and the height of the column rises.

In the setting of myocardial infarction (MI) tachycardia indicates incipient or overt CHF.

The rapid heart rate responds to treatment of heart failure.

Dyspnea on exertion suggests heart failure; dyspnea at rest suggests pulmonary disease.

Exertion demands an increase in cardiac output. The failing heart does not have the requisite reserve to address the increased requirement and the resulting pulmonary congestion is sensed as dyspnea.

Paroxysmal nocturnal dyspnea (PND), when classic, indicates left heart failure.

PND refers to an awakening from sleep after 2 hours with shortness of breath. The patient gets up, walks about, sometimes to an open window, and frequently spends the rest of the night in a chair.

The pathophysiology is simple: reabsorption of edema fluid that has accumulated in the interstitium of the lower limbs into the circulation produces an endogenous volume load on the left ventricle. Orthopnea, although an important sign of CHF since the increased venous return produced by recumbency is an immediate fluid challenge that precipitates pulmonary congestion, is less specific than PND because the mechanics of breathing are easier in the upright position, and a variety of other diseases that elevate the diaphragm or effect lung function in the supine position result in orthopnea.

The cause of bilateral pleural effusions is almost always CHF.

CHF may cause a unilateral right pleural effusion; a unilateral left-sided effusion should never be ascribed to CHF until all other potential causes are eliminated.

Right-sided pleural effusions in heart failure may reflect the fact that patients with cardiomegaly sleep right side down in order to avoid the sensation of the cardiac impulse transmitted through the pillow. This dependent position during sleep may foster fluid accumulation in the right pleural space.

🔵 Edema in CHF has both a forward (diminished renal perfusion) and backward (increased venous pressure) component.

Decreased renal blood flow activates the renin–angiotensin–aldosterone system (RAAS), thereby enhancing water and salt retention.

🔵 Dilutional hyponatremia is a frequent concomitant of CHF since the diminished renal blood flow prevents a water diuresis in the presence of hypotonicity. Angiotensin II, elevated in CHF, also stimulates central thirst receptors and increases water intake.

Antagonism of the RAAS thus plays an important role in the treatment of CHF. Improving cardiac compensation with diuresis is an effective treatment for the hyponatremia that accompanies CHF.

🔵 The left ventricle tolerates a pressure load well but a volume load poorly; the right ventricle tolerates a volume load well but a pressure load poorly.

The relative wall thickness and difference in compliance of each ventricle is the likely cause of this well-established clinical observation. Thus, the thinner and more compliant right ventricle accommodates moderate left to right shunts well for long periods of time but decompensates rapidly in the face of pulmonary hypertension. The left ventricle by contrast tolerates systemic hypertension or aortic stenosis (AS) well for long periods of time but decompensates more readily in the face of volume loads like that imposed by aortic regurgitation (AR).

🔵 The most common cause of right heart failure is left heart failure.

This truism, usually explained by the facile euphemism "pressure backup," obscures the underlying physiology by implying that the increased left-sided pressures are directly transmitted to the pulmonary arterial system resulting in pulmonary hypertension and right-sided failure. A moment's reflection will dispel this impossibly naive notion: if pulmonary venous pressure rose to the level of the pulmonary artery all cardiopulmonary circulation would stop (blood flows down a pressure gradient) and the patient would die in pulmonary edema. So what mediates the development of pulmonary arterial hypertension when left-sided pressures rise?

🔵 A series of poorly characterized, neural, and possibly humoral, factors, recruited by a rise in left atrial and pulmonary venous pressures, result in pulmonary artery vasoconstriction which limits blood flow into the lungs and protects against pulmonary congestion. The price to pay is a decrease in cardiac output and the imposition of a pressure load on the right ventricle (Fig. 4-1).

Every compensatory mechanism exacts a price; in this case, decreasing pulmonary blood flow limits cardiac output and imposes a load on the right ventricle that presages the development of right heart failure.

First recognized in the setting of mitral stenosis (MS), these reflex changes prevent pulmonary edema, but impose a pressure burden on the right ventricle

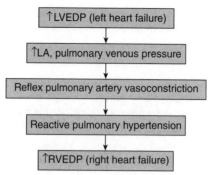

FIGURE 4.1   Left heart failure causes right heart failure. Elevation in left ventricular end diastolic pressure (LVEDP) results in increased left atrial and pulmonary venous pressures which triggers a reflex increase in pulmonary vascular resistance and a rise in pulmonary artery pressure. The pressure load on the right ventricle causes right ventricular failure.

which ultimately fails, since, as noted above, the right ventricle tolerates a pressure load poorly.

The fact that the pulmonary hypertension is rapidly reversed by effective treatment of left heart failure demonstrates that pulmonary vasoconstriction, rather than pulmonary artery remodeling, is responsible.

- **The degree of pulmonary vasoconstriction as a consequence of left heart failure varies in different patients; those with prominent vasoconstrictive responses suffer from reduced cardiac output and, eventually, right heart failure. Those with less pulmonary vasoconstriction develop pulmonary congestion and outright pulmonary edema with less manifestations of right heart failure.**

These series of changes occur with either diastolic (poor ventricular compliance) or systolic dysfunction (low ejection fraction) since both result in a rise in left-sided end diastolic pressures.

- **Hypoxemia, an important cause of pulmonary vasoconstriction, is not the cause of the rise in pulmonary artery pressure that occurs in the setting of left heart failure.**

The mediators of pulmonary vascular tone, in addition to oxygen, include endothelin, nitric oxide, and prostacyclin; how these are regulated in CHF remains uncertain. It is a *faux pearl* that hypoxia mediates the pulmonary artery vasoconstriction that accompanies left heart failure.

- **Left atrial contraction, the so-called "atrial kick," provides a given degree of ventricular stretch at a lower mean left atrial pressure than could be obtained by passive filling of the left ventricle; but for this extra stretch provided at a lower atrial pressure, pulmonary venous pressure would rise, threatening pulmonary edema.**

The importance of atrial contraction depends upon the Frank–Starling law which relates the force of myocardial contraction to diastolic myocardial fiber length: the more stretch, the greater the force of contraction. The increase in stroke volume that accompanies an increase in venous return depends on this mechanism, which also comes into play when diastolic volume is increased in heart failure. To gain the same amount of ventricular stretch without a left atrial kick would require higher left atrial pressures.

> The significance of the atrial kick is clearly demonstrated when a patient with AS develops atrial fibrillation.

Decompensated CHF is the usual result. Rapid rate with diminished time for diastolic filling also contributes importantly.

> Cardiac dilatation has important adverse effects; although dilatation may be viewed as a compensatory mechanism in the face of increased end diastolic pressure, the potential benefit occurs only up to a point.

When overstretched the cardiac myocytes lose their mechanical efficiency and contract poorly. Under these circumstances the cardiac contractility declines, rather than increases, with further stretch (the so-called descending limb of Starling's curve).

> Cardiac dilatation is detrimental for other reasons as well: increased ventricular diameter increases myocardial wall tension (Laplace's law), and wall tension is a major determinant of myocardial oxygen consumption, thus threatening ischemia; and ventricular dilatation alters the spatial relationship of the papillary muscles to each other, so that papillary muscles no longer pull the mitral valve leaflets together resulting in mitral regurgitation (MR).

CHF and Pregnancy

> The absence of CHF symptoms during pregnancy provides historical evidence of adequate cardiac reserve at that time.

Pregnancy history is important in assessing cardiac function. The 30% to 40% increase in plasma volume and cardiac output that peaks early in the third trimester provides a convenient landmark of cardiac reserve at that point in time. This is particularly important in assessing the functional significance of congenital and rheumatic valvular cardiac lesions which may become symptomatic for the first time during pregnancy.

> Peripartum cardiomyopathy is an uncommon cause of CHF occurring late in pregnancy, or more commonly, in the months immediately postpartum.

A dilated cardiomyopathy of unknown cause, the diagnosis of peripartum cardiomyopathy, depends on excluding all other known causes of CHF.

CARDIAC ISCHEMIA

Chest Pain

That chest pain is the hallmark of myocardial ischemia is, of course, well known. The pain is substernal, radiating to the shoulder, left arm, or jaw, frequently with sweating, and, in the presence of MI, associated with a sense of impending doom.

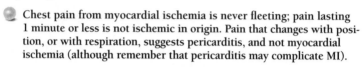 **Chest pain from myocardial ischemia is never fleeting; pain lasting 1 minute or less is not ischemic in origin. Pain that changes with position, or with respiration, suggests pericarditis, and not myocardial ischemia (although remember that pericarditis may complicate MI).**

Myocardial Ischemia and Infarction

The determinants of myocardial oxygen consumption (MVO_2) are heart rate, contractile state, and ventricular wall tension. Since tension is proportional to intraventricular pressure and ventricular radius (Laplace's law), diastolic volume of the heart is directly related to MVO_2.

SNS stimulation increases all of these determinants, save ventricular diameter, providing the physiologic basis for the clinically established role of β-blockade in the treatment and prophylaxis of myocardial ischemia.

Ischemia may result from diminished oxygen supply or increased demand, or both. Decreased supply occurs with the abrupt narrowing or closure of a coronary vessel while increased demand results from increases in the determinants of MVO_2: tachycardia, increased BP, and/or an increase in ventricular volume.

MI may be transmural or subendocardial. Q waves and ST segment elevation suggest transmural infarction from an abrupt change in supply; subendocardial infarction is associated with ST segment depression in the leads reflecting the ischemic area.

Subendocardial ischemia is most common in situations of increased demand because of the unique vulnerability of the subendocardium to alterations in perfusion.

This vulnerability depends on the facts that the subendocardium resides at the distal end of the coronary circulation, and that it is subject to the highest wall pressure by virtue of its location next to the high-pressure ventricular cavity.

Although usually associated with plaque rupture and acute coronary occlusion, transmural infarction may also occur with coronary vasospasm.

Vasospasm may occur with completely normal coronaries or in association with atherosclerotic changes.

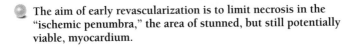 The aim of early revascularization is to limit necrosis in the "ischemic penumbra," the area of stunned, but still potentially viable, myocardium.

PERICARDITIS

Acute Pericarditis

Acute pericarditis has many potential causes, but most often no etiology can be established resulting in the designation "idiopathic." Most of these idiopathic cases are secondary to systemic viral infections (coxsackie or other enteroviruses). Pericarditis may also complicate intrathoracic infections with bacteria or fungi, tuberculosis being a classic example. Collagen vascular disease, post-MI, uremia, and metastatic malignancy are other possible causes.

The pain of pericarditis is accentuated by deep breathing and cough, worse on lying supine, and ameliorated by sitting up.

Diagnosis is secured by a friction rub and characteristic EKG changes. The rub may be brought out on examination by having the patient lean forward or kneel on all fours with the stethoscope held on the precordium. The EKG shows widespread ST elevations that often evolve into T wave inversions, PR depression, and, in the presence of a significant pericardial effusion, electrical alternans, a beat-to beat-variation in the height of the R wave as the heart swings in the fluid-filled pericardial sac.

The feared complication of pericarditis, pericardial tamponade is suggested on physical examination (PE) and confirmed by echocardiography.

Pulsus paradoxus (10 mm Hg drop on inspiration), absent point of maximal impulse (PMI), distant heart sounds, and jugular venous distention (JVD) suggest the diagnosis. Cardiac echo shows fluid accumulation and collapse of the right ventricle, an indication for immediate pericardiocentesis.

Pericarditis may be associated with MI in the immediate postinfarct period or following the infarction by weeks to months (Dressler's syndrome). The incidence of both types of pericarditis has diminished substantially in recent years due to revascularization in the treatment of the acute event, presumably by limiting infarct size.

Peri-infarction pericarditis is caused by pericardial inflammation from contiguous necrotic myocardium. Almost always benign and self-limited, a developing pericardial effusion post MI is nonetheless grounds for discontinuing anticoagulation.

Dressler's syndrome (post-MI syndrome) is an autoimmune reaction that also occurs in postsurgical patients (the postcardiotomy syndrome). Anti-inflammatory agents are useful for symptomatic control.

Chronic Constrictive Pericarditis

Chronic pericardial constriction limits the filling of all cardiac chambers and produces changes suggesting CHF.

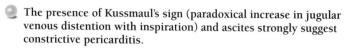 **The presence of Kussmaul's sign (paradoxical increase in jugular venous distention with inspiration) and ascites strongly suggest constrictive pericarditis.**

The causes of constrictive pericarditis include indolent infection (TB, fungi), malignant infiltration, collagen vascular disease, irradiation, and in many cases, unknown.

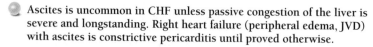 **Ascites is uncommon in CHF unless passive congestion of the liver is severe and longstanding. Right heart failure (peripheral edema, JVD) with ascites is constrictive pericarditis until proved otherwise.**

The cause of the ascites is obscure but may reflect lymphatic obstruction at the level of the liver.

Diagnosis of pericardial constriction may be difficult since imaging is frequently inconclusive; pericardial calcification is highly suggestive.

In addition to Kussmaul's sign a pericardial knock (accentuated third heart sound) may be heard. Right heart catheterization is usually required to demonstrate equalization of pressures in all four cardiac chambers and the pulmonary artery. Despite the high left-sided pressures pulmonary hypertension does not occur.

VALVULAR CARDIAC LESIONS

With the striking diminution in acute rheumatic fever the spectrum of valvular lesions has changed. MS is much less common as are combinations of lesions that used to affect several valves.

The so-called "functional murmur," which is not reflective of cardiac valvular disease, is a flow murmur usually originating over the pulmonic valve and heard best to the left of the sternum in the second intercostal space.

The murmur is accentuated by situations in which the cardiac output is increased such as fever, pregnancy, and thyrotoxicosis.

Aortic Stenosis

Lone AS in the sixth decade of life is most commonly associated with congenital bicuspid valves which calcify early; in the seventh decade and above atherosclerotic calcific AS in a tricuspid aortic valve is the most common cause of AS.

The well-known characteristic murmur of AS is harsh, located at the upper right sternal border, crescendo-decrescendo, and transmitted up the carotids and the subclavian vessels. The murmur may be present in the absence of significant obstruction (calcific aortic sclerosis). The challenge is determining, from the physical examination, whether there is significant stenosis that is associated with a substantial, hemodynamically significant, gradient across the valve.

The most useful physical findings that suggest hemodynamically significant AS are a quiet to absent aortic closure sound (S_2), a pulse delay with a slow upstroke at the carotid artery, and a late peaking murmur.

The left ventricle tolerates the pressure load from significant AS for substantial periods of time. Once symptoms occur the course is rapidly downhill.

The classic symptom triad of AS is well known: angina, syncope, and CHF. The appearance of any of these heralds the need for subsequent evaluation and likely valve replacement.

There is no medical treatment for AS.

AS is the one situation in which the cardiac output increases immediately after open heart surgery.

Syncope in AS results from exercise-induced vasodilation in the setting of a fixed cardiac output due to the stenotic valve. CHF manifests as exertional dyspnea due to diastolic dysfunction.

Although elderly patients with AS frequently have coexisting coronary artery disease, angina may occur with AS in the absence of coronary disease.

The thickened myocardium and the high intraventricular pressures in AS compromise subendocardial blood flow so that oxygen delivery cannot meet the demand imposed by exertion.

Aortic Regurgitation

Chronic AR may be due to valvular disease or, more commonly, disease of the aortic root with dilatation and stretching of the aortic annulus.

Aortic root dilatation occurs with aortic aneurysms, dissections, severe hypertension, or cystic medial necrosis of the aorta.

The latter is the lesion of Marfan's syndrome, but also occurs without the other Marfan's stigmata.

The ascultatory findings are different in valvular AR as compared with AR secondary to root dilatation. In valvular AR the aortic closure sound is usually muted and the regurgitant decrescendo murmur loudest at the left sternal border; in root disease the aortic closure sound is accentuated and may be booming while the murmur is loudest at the upper right sternal border.

The "tambour" sign of aortic valve closure was classically described in syphilitic aortic aneurysm.

- **The peripheral signs of AR reflect the large pulse pressure and depend upon the size of the regurgitant jet.**

- **The water hammer (Corrigan's or Watson's) pulse with a rapid upswing and collapsing downswing is the easiest sign to elicit.**

The water hammer pulse is recognized by holding the patient's forearm upright and squeezing; when a clear pulse is felt the test is positive.

- **In AR the precordium is active, reflecting the increased ventricular volume, while in AS the precordium is quiet.**

In both AR and AS, left ventricular hypertrophy (LVH) is indicated by an abnormally sustained PMI; eventually, lateral displacement of the PMI occurs.

- **Although chronic AR, which develops slowly, may be tolerated for significant periods of time by the gradual increase in ventricular compliance, acute AR is a medical emergency that requires immediate intervention.**

- **The major causes of acute AR are valve rupture from acute bacterial endocarditis and dissecting aneurysm of aorta.**

Trauma to the chest is another cause.

Mitral Stenosis

- **MS and MR, in times past, were common manifestations of rheumatic heart disease. The valves themselves, inflamed by rheumatic fever, became fused in either a stenotic or open position, or commonly both.**

New cases of MS are now very uncommon.

- **A tipoff to the diagnosis of MS is a booming first heart sound, much easier to recognize than the classic diastolic rumble.**

- **The symptoms of MS reflect either low cardiac output or pulmonary congestion.**

As left atrial pressure and pulmonary venous pressure rise pulmonary congestion and/or pulmonary hypertension develop. Depending on the degree of pulmonary hypertension, which diminishes pulmonary blood flow, either recurrent bouts of pulmonary edema or low cardiac output with right heart failure dominate the clinical picture.

- **MS is classically associated with atrial fibrillation and pulmonary hypertension.**

One of the observations in the early days of mitral valvulotomy, contrary to expectation, was that the pulmonary hypertension usually reversed but the atrial fibrillation did not.

Mitral Regurgitation

MR is quite common and has a diverse set of causes.

- The major current causes of MR are ischemic heart disease with papillary muscle infarction and rupture; left ventricular dilatation with distortion of the spatial relationship of the papillary muscles to each other so that contraction does not result in valve closure; mitral valve prolapse (MVP); and, in the elderly, calcification of the mitral annulus.

- The murmur of MR is pansystolic, obliterates S_2, and radiates to the axilla.

- MR remains a significant risk for the development of subacute bacterial endocarditis.

- Chronic MR is better tolerated than chronic AR because there is less cardiac dilatation.

In chronic MR the low-pressure runoff into the compliant left atrium allows the left ventricular volume to diminish during systole; in chronic AR the ventricle expands during diastole because of the volume load created by the regurgitant jet from the high-pressure aorta, and cannot shrink much during systole because it is pumping into the high-pressure circuit. As a consequence the volume increases in the left ventricle are much greater with AR as compared with MR, and the adverse effects of cardiac dilatation outlined above come into play.

- Afterload reduction is an effective treatment for MR since it increases the fraction of the ventricular ejection that flows forward.

- Acute MR, in distinction to the chronic situation, results in immediate severe pulmonary edema.

In acute MR, as occurs with papillary muscle rupture, the relatively noncompliant left atrium does not accommodate the regurgitant jet well, so that left atrial pressures rise dramatically and pulmonary edema ensues.

- Rupture of a chordae tendinae produces a high-pitched whiff of MR; since the regurgitant jet is much smaller, chordae tendinae ruptures are much better tolerated than papillary muscle ruptures.

Both papillary muscle rupture and ruptured chordae may complicate MI.

- MVP is diagnosed by maneuvers that rapidly decrease venous return, such as standing the patient up while listening over the left lower precordium; a midsystolic click and/or a murmur of MR suggest the diagnosis which can be confirmed by echocardiography.

MVP, also known as the "billowing mitral valve" or Barlow's syndrome, is caused by myxomatous degeneration of the mitral valve leaflets.

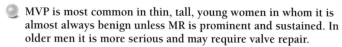

- MVP is most common in thin, tall, young women in whom it is almost always benign unless MR is prominent and sustained. In older men it is more serious and may require valve repair.

- The cause of MVP is unknown in most instances although it is sometimes associated with pectus excavatum and scoliosis. It also occurs in connective tissue diseases such as the Marfan or Ehler–Danlos syndrome.

If MR is present antibiotic prophylaxis for dental procedures is recommended.

Tricuspid Regurgitation

- Tricuspid regurgitation is almost always a consequence of pulmonary hypertension which dilates the right ventricle and stretches the annulus. Since the usual cause is left heart failure the treatment is aimed at relief of CHF; diuresis is usually effective and surgery is rarely required.

The carcinoid syndrome and various congenital cardiac lesions may also be associated with tricuspid regurgitation.

LEFT VENTRICULAR HYPERTROPHY (LVH) AND HYPERTROPHIC CARDIOMYOPATHY (HCM)

The usual cause of LVH is increased afterload from hypertension or AS. In HCM LVH occurs without an increase in afterload.

- In LVH the PMI is sustained and displaced laterally. A fourth heart sound and left atrial enlargement on EKG are early signs of LVH.

HCM is a genetic abnormality in a sarcomeric protein that causes hypertrophy and disarray of cardiomyocyte architecture.

- Asymmetric septal hypertrophy may occur as part of HCM. Contraction of the septum may cause outflow tract obstruction, also referred to as subaortic stenosis.

It is possible to distinguish outflow tract obstruction from valvular AS on PE. The aortic closure sound is not muffled and the pulse is bifid rather than plateau in outflow tract as compared with valvular obstruction; the murmur in outflow tract obstruction is loudest at the lower left sternal border and not the classic aortic area at the upper right sternal border.

- MR is frequently associated with septal hypertrophy.

The characteristic murmur can be heard in the axilla.

- HCM is the leading cause of sudden death in young men.

Affecting athletes in particular, ventricular cardiac arrhythmias are responsible.

🔵 **In the presence of asymmetric septal hypertrophy large septal Q waves on the EKG may be mistaken for evidence of MI.**

Infiltrative diseases affecting the myocardium may also cause the "pseudo infarction" pattern.

CONGENITAL HEART DISEASE IN ADULTS

🔵 **Ostium secundum, the most common form of atrial septal defect (ASD), is frequently diagnosed in young adults. The left to right shunt, if of sufficient size, causes diastolic overload of the right ventricle.**

Exertional dyspnea, fatigue, and increased susceptibility to pulmonary infection are common manifestations.

🔵 **The physical findings are classic and include a fixed split of S_2, a split M_1, a systolic ejection murmur over the pulmonic valve at the upper left sternal border, and a parasternal lift indicative of right ventricular enlargement.**

The left ventricle is small and the PMI is absent.

🔵 **The much less common ostium primum defect, also known as an endocardial cushion defect, is located lower down on the septum; MR is frequently associated.**

🔵 **Chest x-ray in patients with ASD shows right ventricular hypertrophy (RVH), pulmonary vascular congestion and plethoric lungs. EKG shows a right bundle branch block (partial or complete). With the primum defect left anterior hemiblock (left axis deviation) is present as well.**

In the fetal circulation the resistance in the pulmonary circulation is very high thus shunting blood from the venous return through the foramen ovale to the left atrium and thus into the systemic circulation for oxygen exchange in the placenta. In the presence of an atrial septal defect the increased pulmonary resistance of the fetal state regresses so that pulmonary artery pressure remains relatively normal into adulthood in most cases. Eventually, the hyperdynamic pulmonary circulation causes pulmonary hypertension which, over time, becomes fixed. In the case of ventricular septal defect (VSD), if sufficiently large, the pulmonary vascular resistance never regresses and pulmonary hypertension is noted earlier in life. In many VSD cases, however, the pulmonary pressure remains normal until the hyperdynamic pulmonary circulation takes its toll (as with ASD).

🔵 **VSD is associated with a coarse, loud, pansystolic murmur at the left sternal border and a palpable thrill is present in almost all cases.**

In distinction to ASD the left ventricular impulse is prominent in patients with VSD unless the defect is very small. A third heart sound may be present due to rapid left ventricular filling.

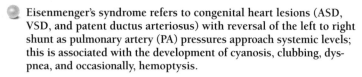

Eisenmenger's syndrome refers to congenital heart lesions (ASD, VSD, and patent ductus arteriosus) with reversal of the left to right shunt as pulmonary artery (PA) pressures approach systemic levels; this is associated with the development of cyanosis, clubbing, dyspnea, and occasionally, hemoptysis.

Described originally with VSD it now includes, prominently, ASD with shunt reversal.

A small VSD ("maladie de Roger") may serve as a nidus for the development of subacute bacterial endocarditis.

Appropriate prophylaxis for dental and other procedures should be considered.

ORTHOSTATIC HYPOTENSION

Orthostatic hypotension is usually defined as an upright fall in systolic BP of 20 mm Hg and a 10 mm Hg fall in diastolic pressure, with symptoms.

Orthostatic hypotension is caused by either a decrease in plasma volume, with its attendant fall in venous return, or by a disruption of the SNS reflexes that normally defend the circulation in the upright position.

Under normal circumstances, standing results in a fall in central venous pressure which initiates a reflex increase in sympathetic nervous system (SNS) outflow to the great veins causing venoconstriction and a corresponding increase in venous return as blood is shifted from the central venous reservoir to the heart. Cardiac output is thereby rapidly restored eliminating a significant fall in BP. Pulse rate may increase as well. Note that this reflex involves the low pressure, capacitance (venous) portion of the circulation; the classic baroreceptors in the high pressure, resistance (arterial) portion of the circulation do not come into play unless there is a fall in arterial BP. The system is designed to prevent an upright fall in BP.

Volume depletion is the most common cause of orthostatic hypotension.

Hemorrhage, vomiting, and diarrhea are the common culprits, along with pharmaceutical agents (diuretics, antihypertensive drugs, and psychotropic agents that antagonize the SNS).

Neurologic diseases or drugs that affect the SNS outflow or the peripheral SNS are also common causes of orthostatic hypertension.

Multiple systems atrophy (Shy–Drager syndrome) is a neurodegenerative disease that affects multiple areas of the central nervous system; Parkinsonian features and orthostatic hypotension are prominent manifestations, the latter a consequence of involvement of the preganglionic sympathetic nerve fibers.

The disease is most common in middle-aged men.

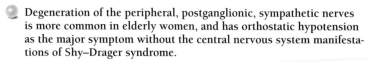 **Degeneration of the peripheral, postganglionic, sympathetic nerves is more common in elderly women, and has orthostatic hypotension as the major symptom without the central nervous system manifestations of Shy–Drager syndrome.**

Since there is no feasible way of restoring the normal relationship between fall in venous return (and fall in BP) and sympathetic activation, treatment is generally ineffective, but measures to expand the plasma volume (high salt diet, fludrocortisone) and to antagonize venous pooling (fitted stockings or pantyhose) offer some relief in mild cases by making the circulation less dependent on SNS reflexes.

In unexplained shock or circulatory collapse, echocardiogram of the right ventricle rapidly distinguishes between hemorrhage and pulmonary embolism; the RV is collapsed in the former and enlarged in the latter.

SYNCOPE

Vasovagal (Neurogenic) Syncope

Syncope, a transient loss of consciousness, is a common occurrence that usually reflects a sudden decrease in cerebral perfusion. The most common cause is a "vasovagal" reaction, also known as neurovascular or neurocardiogenic syncope.

The cause of vasovagal syncope is an abrupt fall in venous return which triggers a paradoxical decrease in SNS tone and an increase in vagal tone with consequent fall in BP, drop in pulse rate, and fall in cardiac output. Certain activities may trigger this response in a reproducible fashion.

The clinical characteristics of a vasovagal faint include a warning aura of lightheadedness, ringing in the ears, nausea, and a slow fall to the ground.

Once the supine position is reached venous return increases and the patient recovers consciousness.

A primitive reflex, evolved in the setting of major trauma with hemorrhage, underlies the vasovagal reaction.

The underlying pathophysiology explains the triggers, the aura, and the clinical features. The usual response to a fall in venous return, as described above, is an increase in SNS activity; when the fall in venous return is abrupt and extreme, however, a primitive reflex comes into play and SNS activity markedly decreases, frequently with an associated increase in vagal tone. In teleologic terms this response would serve several useful functions in the face of severe injury such as major trauma or hemorrhage. The fall in blood pressure would limit bleeding; the decrease in metabolic rate associated with SNS suppression would conserve resources for recovery.

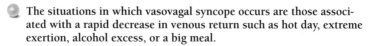 **The situations in which vasovagal syncope occurs are those associated with a rapid decrease in venous return such as hot day, extreme exertion, alcohol excess, or a big meal.**

Interestingly, some people faint at the sight of their own blood as in medical phlebotomy; this may be a CNS (cortical) representation of severe injury that elicits the same primitive response that evolved in the setting of severe trauma with bleeding.

The fall in cerebral perfusion causes the ringing in the ears and dizziness that herald the faint.

The fall in BP is gradual enough that the patient usually slumps down to the supine position without serious injury.

If the cerebral ischemia is more profound or prolonged, seizures may ensue (convulsive syncope). These are usually in the form of myoclonic jerks that are short lived.

Seizures may, of course, also be the cause of syncope.

An elevated prolactin level frequently accompanies seizures and may be useful in reconstructing the episode if blood is available from the time of the attack. Elevation of prolactin level may also occur after some vasovagal episodes.

Although vasovagal syncope is sometimes called neurocardiogenic syncope the heart is not the culprit in this type of fainting and cardiac pacing is of no avail.

Cardiac Syncope

Cardiac syncope is the consequence of a sudden fall in cardiac output due to valvular heart disease (particularly AS), or due to serious disturbance of cardiac rhythm.

Either tachy or brady arrhythmias may be associated with syncope. If the rate is rapid incomplete ventricular filling (shortened diastole) is the cause; in slow rhythms (heart block) rate-related fall in cardiac output is responsible. In AS the outflow across the aortic valve is fixed so that a fall in peripheral resistance with exercise or a decrease in cardiac filling with an increase in heart rate results in a profound fall in cardiac output and a decrease in cerebral perfusion.

In cardiac syncope loss of consciousness is sudden and damage from the fall is much more likely than with the vasovagal reaction. Aura is usually absent.

Head injury from a sudden fall without warning is frequently the clue that the syncope is of cardiac origin.

🔵 **EKG harbingers of complete heart block are important to recognize in patients with syncope since they indicate the need for prompt placement of a cardiac pacemaker.**

EKG characteristics of impending heart block include wide bundle branch block (longer than 0.12, especially if longer than 0.16), bifascicular block (such as right bundle branch block with left anterior hemiblock), and evidence of bilateral bundle branch block (left or right bundle with prolonged PR interval) and alternating bundle branch block showing a left bundle pattern in the standard leads and a right bundle pattern in the precordial leads.

🔵 **A patient presenting with a history of syncope, a bruise about the head, and EKG features suggesting bilateral bundle branch block is a candidate for immediate cardiac pacing.**

Hypertension 5

ESSENTIAL HYPERTENSION

Hypertension is the most important risk factor for stroke and congestive heart failure (CHF), and an important contributor to the risk of
myocardial infarction.

The cardiovascular risk imposed by high blood pressure is reversed toward
normal by effective treatment, with the most improvement in risk of stroke,
and less, but significant risk reduction for myocardial infarction.

The majority of cases of "essential" hypertension occur in association
with obesity.

Up to 70% of essential hypertension may be attributed to obesity. Obesity-
related hypertension is salt sensitive and is associated with insulin resistance
and hyperinsulinemia, sympathetic stimulation secondary to elevated levels of
insulin and leptin, and activation of the renin-angiotensin-aldosterone system
(RAAS). The RAAS activation is at least in part due to synthesis of RAAS components in visceral adipose tissue and release of these components into the
circulation.

The Pressure–Natriuresis Relationship

Blood pressure and sodium excretion are inextricably related. Indeed, the
pathophysiology of hypertension can only be understood in relation to sodium
excretion. As the blood pressure increases, all other things being equal, sodium
excretion increases: this is known as the "pressure–natriuresis relationship,"
described in detail by physiologist Arthur Guyton and his colleagues over five
decades ago. Since the kidney has an infinite capacity to compensate for BP
elevations by increasing salt and water excretion, it follows that the kidney
plays a critical role in the initiation and maintenance of hypertension.

Strong experimental evidence in support of the role of the kidneys in the pathogenesis and maintenance of hypertension includes the fact that norepinephrine (NE), infused intravenously, induces only transient increase in BP; natriuresis ensues with normalization of the BP. Sustained hypertension, on the other hand, results if the same dose of NE is infused into the renal artery, increasing sodium reabsorption and blunting natriuresis.

> **The presence of high blood pressure is always associated with an alteration in the capacity of the kidney to excrete salt, imposing a so-called "natriuretic handicap."**

In the hypertensive state the pressure–natriuresis relationship is shifted to the right: a given amount of sodium excretion is associated with a higher blood pressure (Fig. 5-1).

> **The "natriuretic handicap" of the hypertensive state explains why all diuretics, regardless of class, are effective antihypertensive agents: they help the kidneys excrete salt, thereby restoring the pressure–natriuresis relationship toward normal.**

There is a natural tendency to confuse the natriuretic handicap with salt and water retention, edema and volume expansion; this is not the case. The elevation in blood pressure is a compensatory mechanism that overcomes the altered sodium excretion in order to prevent volume expansion.

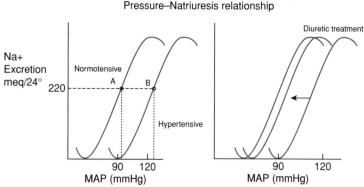

FIGURE 5.1   The pressure–natriuresis relationship: sodium excretion in relation to blood pressure. In balance on a normal sodium intake (say 220 mEq as shown in the figure) the normotensive individual will excrete the day's intake at a mean arterial pressure (MAP) of 90 mm Hg (point A); the hypertensive individual will be able to maintain sodium balance only at a MAP of over 120 mm Hg (point B). This impediment to sodium excretion has been called the "natriuretic handicap" of hypertension. Diuretic treatment helps the kidney excrete salt, thereby moving the pressure natriuresis curve toward normal and addressing the natriuretic handicap.

Despite the natriuretic handicap of hypertension edema and volume expansion are not present because the elevated BP compensates for the renal sodium avidity and permits the maintenance of sodium balance and a normal plasma volume.

The natriuretic handicap of hypertension is best understood in a physiologic context. Precise regulation of blood pressure around a "normal" value is not a high priority. Maintenance of an adequate circulation, critical organ perfusion, and normal plasma volume are high priorities. Unlike serum sodium, or pH, or tonicity, BP varies considerably throughout the day under normal circumstances. BP increases with exercise and falls during sleep, for example. High blood pressure is a long-term, but not a short-term risk, while plasma volume regulation requires precise short-term regulation. A small mismatch in sodium intake and excretion may be fatal, resulting either in shock or pulmonary edema.

High blood pressure, therefore, represents the triumph of volume over pressure in physiologic regulation of the circulation, an example of the "wisdom of the body" to use the phrase coined by Walter Cannon. High blood pressure enables the individual to excrete the day's sodium intake and maintain sodium balance despite an increased renal avidity for sodium.

Hypertension is the footprint of mechanisms evolved to survive trauma, hemorrhage, and extracellular volume depletion.

Essential hypertension may be seen in evolutionary terms as a consequence of mechanisms evolved to maintain an adequate circulation in the face of trauma with blood loss, or in other situations associated with extracellular fluid volume depletion. Such mechanisms include the RAAS and the sympathetic nervous system (SNS), both of which play a role in the maintenance of blood pressure under situations of blood loss or volume depletion as well as in the initiation and maintenance of hypertension. When activated these systems result in vasoconstriction and renal sodium reabsorption. Those individuals on the higher end of the spectrum of activity in these systems would have increased survival in the face of circulatory challenge, a clear short-term survival advantage, but would be predisposed to hypertension and its consequences in the long term.

Most cases of "resistant" hypertension are due to insufficient diuretic inclusion in the regimen.

MALIGNANT HYPERTENSION

In times past much was made of the distinction between "benign" and "malignant" hypertension. The development of highly effective antihypertensive drugs, along with the recognition that "benign" is an inappropriate descriptor for hypertension, has almost, but not completely, rendered these terms of historical interest. It remains of clinical importance to recognize and treat malignant hypertension aggressively.

🟢 Malignant hypertension is a medical emergency that requires prompt evaluation and treatment.

Unrecognized and untreated treated malignant hypertension is usually lethal within a year.

🟢 The pathologic hallmark of malignant hypertension is fibrinoid arteriolar necrosis. Clinical evidence of the latter may be found in the eye grounds and in the urine.

On funduscopic examination, flame-shaped hemorrhages and "cotton-wool" spots (fluffy exudates), which signify retinal infarction, are diagnostic of malignant hypertension. Papilledema, due to ischemia of the nerve head or increased intracranial pressure, often in association with hypertensive encephalopathy, are also indicative of malignant hypertension. Damage to the kidney is assessed by the urine analysis: heavy proteinuria and hematuria are consistent with malignant hypertension.

🟢 Malignant hypertension is much more common in current smokers.

Prompt lowering of the BP is essential to limit and reverse end organ damage.

🟢 Malignant hypertension requires the consideration and the exclusion of secondary causes, particularly renal artery stenosis (RAS) and pheochromocytoma.

SECONDARY HYPERTENSION

🟢 Secondary causes should be ruled out when the hypertension is severe, when it occurs in the young, or when the onset is abrupt.

Particular attention should be directed to the correctible secondary causes including coarctation of the aorta, RAS, primary hyperaldosteronism, pheochromocytoma, and rarely, Cushing's syndrome (Table 5-1).

🟢 Coarctation of the aorta, has a strong male predominance, is diagnosed by a delay in the femoral pulse, is frequently associated with a bicuspid aortic valve, and when noted in a female, Turner's syndrome is likely.

🟢 It is a *faux pearl* that hyperthyroidism and the carcinoid syndrome are causes of secondary hypertension.

Hyperthyroidism is associated with an increase in cardiac output and a wide pulse pressure; the diastolic BP is decreased. The carcinoid syndrome is associated with kinin-mediated hypotension rather than serotonin-mediated hypertension.

Renal Artery Stenosis

🟢 The hypertension of RAS is usually severe and may be accentuated or brought on by oral contraceptives.

TABLE 5.1 Correctable Secondary Hypertension

Disease	Screening Test	Diagnostic Test	Treatment
Coarctation of aorta	Femoral pulse delay	Imaging	Surgery
Renal artery stenosis	Abdominal bruit RA Doppler	Imaging; renal vein renin	Angioplasty; stent; surgery; medication
Primary aldosteronism	Suppressed plasma renin; increased plasma aldosterone	Adrenal vein catheterization	Surgery; spironolactone
Pheochromocytoma	Symptoms; plasma metanephrines	24-hour urinary catecholamines and metanephrines; imaging	Alpha blockade; surgery
Cushing's syndrome	Overnight dexamethasone suppression test	24-hour urinary cortisol; imaging	Surgery

● A young Caucasian hypertensive woman with a flame hemorrhage in the eye grounds has a greater than 50% chance of having RAS.

● RAS is the most common correctable secondary cause of hypertension. In young women fibromuscular hyperplasia with a beaded appearance of the renal artery is the usual cause.

Frequent pregnancies may predispose to this lesion and the right renal artery is most commonly affected, perhaps because of its longer intra-abdominal course and the tension exerted on this artery by a gravid uterus. The diagnosis is suggested by the appropriate history supported by a bruit on physical examination, a smaller kidney on the affected side, and is diagnosed by imaging of the vessels.

● The hemodynamic significance of RAS is assessed by catheterization of the renal veins and demonstration of a step-up of renin on the affected side.

Angioplasty of the affected artery in cases of fibromuscular hyperplasia is usually of significant benefit.

● In the elderly atherosclerotic obstruction at the take off of the renal arteries is the most common form of RAS.

It should be suspected when patients with peripheral vascular disease have an accentuation of their hypertension and are less responsive to antihypertensive drugs.

Primary Aldosteronism

Primary aldosteronism (PA) is a relatively common cause of second-ary hypertension, but the true incidence is the subject of intense current debate.

After RAS PA is probably the most common cause of secondary hypertension. Hypokalemia in a patient not on diuretics suggests the diagnosis, but it is now recognized that many patients have normal serum potassium levels, especially if on a low salt diet. The diagnosis is confirmed by demonstrating a suppressed plasma renin and an elevated plasma aldosterone level.

Since potassium influences aldosterone secretion the testing for PA should be done in a potassium replete state. Low potassium levels will falsely lower aldosterone levels.

The much more common secondary aldosteronism is easily distin-guished from the primary form by a high plasma renin level.

Once the diagnosis of primary hyperaldosteronism is made the cause needs to be established. Is it a unilateral adenoma (classic Conn's tumor), or bilateral adrenal hyperplasia?

The distinction is important because the adenoma is cured by surgery, but not the hyperplasia. Even bilateral adrenalectomy does not cure the hypertension in hyper-plasia cases, for reasons that remain obscure. Unfortunately, the distinction cannot be made reliably by imaging; many aldosterone-secreting adenomas are small and below the resolution of current clinical imaging techniques. The issue is resolved by simultaneous sampling of the adrenal veins for aldosterone and cortisol. The right adrenal vein comes off the vena cava at a 90-degree angle, is difficult to can-nulate, and is subject to more dilution with caval blood than the left adrenal vein which arises from the left renal vein, has a long course, is easy to cannulate, and less subject to systemic dilution. Cortisol corrects for the dilution problem. The ratio of aldosterone to cortisol on each side is compared and a significant step up on one side, with systemic levels on the other, localizes the lesion. Simultaneous draws (not sequential) are required since adrenocorticotropic hormone (ACTH) fluctu-ates widely even over brief periods of time and will change the adrenal venous cortisol levels, thereby altering the denominator in the aldosterone cortisol ratio. This may affect the results if the draws are performed sequentially.

Normalization of the BP on spironolactone predicts a good BP response to adrenalectomy in patients with PA.

A trial of spironolactone can be undertaken while awaiting the results of the adrenal venous sampling. In bilateral hyperplasia cases spironolactone corrects the hypokalemia but does not normalize the blood pressure.

Pheochromocytoma

🔵 Although an uncommon cause of hypertension, many cases of pheo-chromocytoma go undiagnosed. The trick is to think of the diagnosis. In the great majority of cases the diagnosis is easily established by plasma metanephrines and/or a 24-hour urine for fractionated cat-echolamines (epinephrine and norepinephrine) and metanephrines.

Unselected autopsy series have shown that the majority of pheochromocyto-mas found at postmortem examination were not diagnosed during life; sub-sequent chart review of these cases demonstrates that in most of them the tumor was the cause of death. Since pheochromocytoma is almost always cur-able when diagnosed, and invariably fatal when not, the premium on prompt recognition is great.

🔵 Common symptoms that should raise the suspicion of pheochromo-cytoma include the well-recognized triad of headache, sweating, and palpitation.

The hypertension in patients with pheochromocytoma is usually sustained but frequently more variable than in essential hypertension. In some patients the hypertension is truly episodic, occurring only during characteristic paroxysms.

🔵 Paroxysms are discrete and episodic lasting from 5 minutes to an hour or more. Headache, sweating, palpitations, and chest or abdom-inal pain are common symptoms associated with the paroxysms.

🔵 Paroxysms may be induced by drugs or medical procedures. Opioids, in particular, cause release of catecholamines from the tumor and may cause a severe or fatal paroxysm.

Fentanyl, given as a preanesthetic medication to patients with unexpected pheochromocytoma, has induced fatal paroxysms on many occasions.

🔵 Any unexpected changes in BP during a medical procedure (up or down), particularly if severe, should raise the suspicion of pheochromocytoma.

🔵 In an untreated hypertensive patient an orthostatic fall in BP should raise the suspicion of pheochromocytoma.

Orthostatic hypotension is common in patients with pheochromocytoma. Decreased plasma volume due to alpha receptor-mediated venoconstriction is the major cause. Venoconstriction shrinks the capacitance portion of the cir-culation. Since the body senses changes in volume by pressure changes in the capacitance central veins, venoconstriction is interpreted as a "full tank" when, in fact, the tank is smaller and has less reserve for defending the blood pressure during orthostatic stress.

🔵 Other less common presentations of pheochromocytoma include unexplained hypotension or shock.

The pathophysiology of a fall in BP likely involves decreased plasma volume from long-standing catecholamine-induced venoconstriction, but the release of hypotensive peptides, such as adrenomedullin, from the tumor may be involved in some of these unusual cases. Shock lung (acute respiratory distress syndrome [ARDS]) may occur and may be the presenting manifestation of a crisis. Catecholamine-induced cardiac fibrosis with CHF is a complication as well.

 The old saw "forget a fat pheo" does not always "cut wood" but is right more often than not, and obese patients with a pheochromocytoma usually have lost weight prior to diagnosis.

Patients with pheochromocytoma have an increase in metabolic rate due to catecholamine stimulation of heat production largely in brown adipose tissue. This increase in thermogenesis does not result in fever unless the capacity of the body to dissipate the excess heat production is exceeded. Nonetheless, heat dissipation by sweating may dominate the clinical picture. The increase in metabolic rate is frequently associated with weight loss in the period leading up to the diagnosis.

 Bilateral adrenal pheochromocytomas are always familial (autosomal dominant inheritance), but a unilateral pheochromocytoma does not rule out an inherited pheochromocytoma or associated syndrome.

Associated syndromes include: MEN 2 A (medullary carcinoma of the thyroid, pheochromocytoma, and hyperparathyroidism); MEN 2B (medullary carcinoma of the thyroid, pheochromocytoma, mucosal neuromas); von Hipple–Lindau (VHL) retinal cerebellar hemangioblastomatosis; von Recklinghausen's neurofibromatosis type 1; familial paraganglioma syndromes (succinic dehydrogenase B [SDHB] mutations).

 Extra-adrenal pheochromocytomas are frequently referred to as paragangliomas, but the latter do not always produce catecholamines, and never produce epinephrine.

The characteristics of pheochromocytoma vary in the different familial syndromes. In both MEN syndromes the pheochromocytomas are multicentric within the adrenals, usually bilateral at presentation, and secreting epinephrine as well as NE. Early on in screening familial cases elevated epinephrine excretion may be the only abnormality. Extra-adrenal pheochromocytomas do not occur as part of the MEN syndromes. With VHL both intra- and extra-adrenal pheochromocytomas are common, the incidence varying greatly in different kindreds depending on the particular genetic mutation. In the familial paraganglioma syndromes both extra-adrenal and adrenal pheochromocytomas may occur. The incidence of malignancy is higher with the SDHB mutations than in sporadic cases.

Perhaps 25% of pheochromocytomas are familial, 75% sporadic, and the incidence of malignancy overall is about 10% (higher in the paraganglioma syndromes).

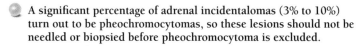 A significant percentage of adrenal incidentalomas (3% to 10%) turn out to be pheochromocytomas, so these lesions should not be needled or biopsied before pheochromocytoma is excluded.

Pheochromocytomas appear characteristically dense on MRI T2-weighted images.

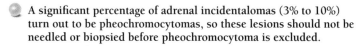 Alpha adrenergic blockade with phenoxybenzamine should be instituted for about 2 weeks before surgical excision; achieving the final dose must be done gradually by titrating the dose to normalize the blood pressure.

The surgery may be performed by a minimally invasive approach, anatomy permitting.

Cushing's Syndrome

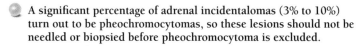 Although most patients with Cushing's syndrome have some of the usual stigmata of glucocorticoid excess, an occasional case, early in the course of disease, may present with hypertension as the major manifestation.

This is particularly true in young women.

Polycystic Kidney Disease (PKD)

Inherited as an autosomal dominant trait (ADPKD), hypertension is an early manifestation of PKD in young adults.

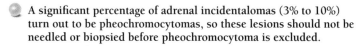 The combination of hypertension, flank pain, hematuria, renal colic (clots), and large tender abdominal masses is diagnostic of PKD.

Although not correctable except by transplantation it is important to recognize this entity. Berry aneurysms in the cerebral circulation are classically associated with PKD, likely because of the long-standing hypertension.

AORTIC DISSECTION

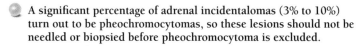 Aortic dissections are of two types depending on the location of the intimal tear: ascending (arch) and descending aorta.

The presenting symptoms and treatment differ substantially (Table 5-2).

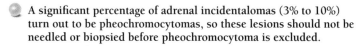 Ascending arch (type A, DeBakey type 1) dissections, the most common type, present with the sudden onset of chest pain and are often followed by syncope and shock; descending aortic dissections (type B, DeBakey type 3) typically present with back pain of a tearing quality, often with a very high blood pressure.

Absent, diminished, or asymmetric peripheral pulses may be noted and the D dimer is frequently elevated due to clot propagation and fibrinolysis in the

TABLE 5.2 Aortic Dissection

Ascending (arch) Dissections	Descending (thoracic) Dissections
Anterior chest pain, syncope, and shock	Pain radiating to the back, severe, "tearing" quality
Confirmed by CT angio, TEE	Confirmed by CT angio, TEE
Complications: acute AR; left-sided hemothorax; cardiac tamponade; carotid, coronary dissection, or occlusion with cerebrovascular accident (CVA) or MI	Complications: renal, mesenteric, spinal, or femoral artery dissection or occlusion
Treatment: immediate surgery	Treatment: antihypertensive meds to decrease dP/dt, lower BP, stop propagation and relieve pain; surgery later, if needed

false lumen. The diagnosis can be confirmed by CT angiogram or transesophageal echocardiography (TEE), both of which permit localization of the intimal tear. The underlying pathology of aortic dissection is cystic medial necrosis, hypertension is the usual predisposing cause, and the possibility of Marfan's or Ehlers–Danlos syndrome should be considered.

 Ascending dissections are frequently complicated by aortic regurgitation and occasionally by left-sided hemothorax or cardiac tamponade; immediate surgical repair is required.

Antihypertensive therapy is rarely indicated in ascending dissections since the patients are usually in shock. Stroke or MI may complicate the picture from compromise of the cerebral or coronary circulations.

 Descending dissections are frequently associated with severe hypertension and need immediate antihypertensive treatment to limit the propagation of the false lumen.

Since propagation depends on the force of ventricular contraction (the "dP/dt") agents with negative inotropic effect are required and should always be administered prior to vasodilators like nitroprusside which cause reflex SNS stimulation. The blood pressure should be lowered until the pain stops. Surgery may be delayed and may not be needed in all cases if the dissection heals with hypotensive therapy.

Branches of the descending aorta may be compromised leading to renal failure and/or spinal cord ischemia from involvement of the spinal arteries.

The Kidney and Disorders of Fluid and Acid–Base Balance

6

CHAPTER

ABNORMAL RENAL FUNCTION TESTS

Bun and Creatinine

When a patient presents with abnormal renal function tests three questions arise: is there a hemodynamic cause?; is urinary tract obstruction present?; is there intrinsic renal disease present, and if so, is this glomerular or interstitial, or primary or secondary?

Volume depletion is the usual hemodynamic cause; decreased renal blood flow with a lesser decrease in glomerular filtration rate (prerenal azotemia) is indicated by a low fractional excretion of sodium. Hemorrhage or extracellular fluid losses from diuretics, vomiting, or diarrhea are the usual culprits.

- The blood urea nitrogen (BUN) is a better indicator of uremic symptoms than the serum creatinine which is a better indicator of glomerular filtration rate (GFR).

- The BUN reflects protein intake, so a patient who has not been eating may have a BUN that is less reflective of renal function.

- In the presence of volume depletion BUN is affected more than serum creatinine since decreased renal blood flow is associated with back diffusion of urea (urea clearance is affected more than creatinine clearance).

The ratio of BUN to creatinine, normally about 10 to 1, is increased in prerenal azotemia.

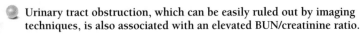 **Urinary tract obstruction, which can be easily ruled out by imaging techniques, is also associated with an elevated BUN/creatinine ratio.**

Plasma Volume Assessment

The clinical assessment of volume status is crucial in the severely ill patient. Neck vein distention 3 cm above the clavicle at 30 degrees of elevation indicates an increased filling pressure. Edema is a critical sign. In a bed-ridden patient edema of the posterior thighs may be more reliable than pedal or pretibial fluid.

Edema always means excess fluid; it equilibrates well and rapidly with the plasma volume.

Exceptions are intense arteriolar vasodilation without venodilation (e.g., calcium channel blockers, cytokine release in septic shock), venous insufficiency, and extremely low albumin levels. With these absent, there is no such thing as "volume depletion" in an edematous patient.

The body assesses volume status from changes in pressure in the capacitance (low pressure) portion of the circulation (great veins and right atrium).

The body is good at assessing changes in pressure but unable to assess changes in volume, so it uses a surrogate to estimate plasma volume based on pressure in the capacitance vessels. A decrease in plasma volume decreases venous return which decreases the pressure (stretch) in the great veins and the right atrium; this decrease in pressure stimulates the sympathetic nervous system causing venoconstriction which returns blood from the periphery to the central venous reservoir, thereby compensating for the volume deficit and maintaining cardiac output. This occurs at the expense of a diminished plasma volume. At the same time activation of the renin-angiotensin-aldosterone system (RAAS) increases renal sodium reabsorption tending to restore extracellular fluid volume.

The entity of "stress polycythemia" is really hemoconcentration around a normal red cell mass.

Conversely, an increase in plasma volume increases the pressure (and stretch) in the capacitance portion of the circulation, diminishes sympathetic activity, suppresses the RAAS, and initiates a diuresis, thereby diminishing the extracellular fluid volume.

HYPONATREMIA

Volume Depletion Hyponatremia

Hyponatremia in the presence of volume depletion represents the triumph of volume over tonicity (Table 6-1).

TABLE 6.1 Hyponatremia

	BUN/ Creatinine	Urinary NA	Plasma Renin, Uric Acid	Treatment
Volume depletion hyponatremia (reset osmoreceptors)	↑	↓	↑	Normal saline
Dilutional hyponatremia (impaired free water clearance) SIADH	↓	↑	↓	Water restriction, 3% saline
CHF	↑	↓	↑	Diuresis
Cirrhosis	−/↑	↓	↑	Diuresis, pressors, albumin

Low-serum sodium is either dilutional or secondary to diminished plasma volume. In the latter, as plasma volume diminishes neural afferent impulses from the low-pressure capacitance portion of the circulation change the normal relationship between tonicity and antidiuretic hormone (ADH) release so that ADH is released at lower plasma tonicity than normal. This represents a resetting of the central osmoreceptors. Volume is thereby preserved at the expense of tonicity.

 In volume depletion hyponatremia the urine is concentrated, the urinary sodium is low, and plasma renin and serum uric acid are high, reflecting diminished renal blood flow.

Volume depletion hyponatremia thus represents the wisdom of the body in defending an adequate circulatory volume at the expense of maintaining normal tonicity. Treatment thus entails volume resuscitation with normal saline that permits a water diuresis and the prompt restitution of the serum sodium.

Dilutional Hyponatremia

 The essential abnormality of dilutional hyponatremia is the inability to have a water diuresis in the presence of an increased extracellular fluid volume and a low plasma tonicity.

Dilutional hyponatremia is complicated in both pathophysiology and treatment.

Syndrome of Inappropriate Secretion of ADH (SIADH)

The purest form of dilutional hypernatremia is the SIADH. The inappropriate ADH may be synthesized and secreted ectopically by tumors (lung or other), released from the posterior pituitary by poorly characterized reflex mechanisms, or result from the action of drugs which potentiate ADH release.

● A very low-serum uric acid may be a tip off to the diagnosis of SIADH.

● Intrathoracic lesions such as pneumonia or CNS lesions such as strokes are common causes of SIADH.

In SIADH the tonicity of urine usually exceeds that of plasma and in all cases is less than maximally dilute. The urinary sodium concentration is high, reflective of the daily salt intake.

● The natriuresis that occurs in SIADH once again represents the triumph of volume over tonicity, since the plasma volume expansion induced by water reabsorption is countered by salt excretion.

In the past this led to the outmoded concepts of "pulmonary" or "cerebral" salt wasting since the high urinary sodium was recognized before the physiology of the dilutional state was understood. The treatment is fluid restriction (below insensible loss) and hypertonic saline if the hyponatremia is severe or symptomatic.

● Other forms of dilutional hyponatremia that may occur with clinically obvious expansion of the extracellular fluid space include congestive heart failure (CHF) and cirrhosis.

In these cases it is likely that a primary decrease in renal blood flow impairs the ability to clear free water. This is supported by a high plasma renin and elevated serum uric acid, both reflections of diminished renal perfusion. Treatment is aimed at restoring renal perfusion so that a water diuresis is possible.

● Thiazide-induced hyponatremia has features of both volume depletion and dilution.

It rapidly normalizes after discontinuation of the thiazide diuretic.

● The hyponatremia of Addison's disease reflects both hypovolemia (deficient aldosterone) and the fact that a permissive level of glucocorticoid is necessary to achieve maximal impermeability of the distal nephron to water in the absence of ADH.

Thus, back diffusion of water limits the ability to clear free water. This explains the hyponatremia of secondary adrenal insufficiency which occurs in spite of unimpaired aldosterone secretion.

Hyponatremia is common in hypopituitarism despite normal aldo-sterone secretion since permissive amounts of glucocorticoids and thyroid hormones are necessary for a normal water diuresis.

URINARY SODIUM AND POTASSIUM

Sodium and Potassium Balance

In the absence of disease a state of sodium and potassium balance exists: excretion reflects dietary intake. Nothing is gained by measur-ing these cations unless you are assessing the renal response to a physiologic perturbation such as hyponatremia or hypokalemia.

In volume depletion, for example, the kidney conserves sodium and the uri-nary sodium will be very low. In dilutional forms of hyponatremia the sodium will be high (reflective of intake).

In patients with hypokalemia a spot urine potassium measurement is very useful: a urinary potassium level below 20 mEq/L suggests extra-renal losses; higher urinary potassium indicates renal loss, usually secondary to increased aldosterone secretion, which induces potassium and hydrogen ion excretion in exchange for sodium reabsorption.

ACID–BASE DISTURBANCES

Metabolic Acidosis

In the absence of toxic ingestion or advanced renal failure an anion gap acidosis is either lactic acidosis or ketoacidosis. If measurements for ketones in the blood are negative, lactic acid is the cause.

The causes of lactic acidosis are many, but poor perfusion and tissue necrosis, often in the setting of multiple organ failure, are frequent contributors. Keto-acidosis is caused by hepatic ketone overproduction, the latter a consequence of insulin deficiency at the level of both the liver and adipose tissue depots throughout the body. Circulating free fatty acids (FFAs) are the substrate for ketone production. Low levels of insulin, as found in the fasting state, encour-age lipolysis in adipose tissue and the increased generation of FFAs. In the liver, the FFAs are converted into ketoacids (β-hydroxybutyrate and acetoacetate) rather than synthesized into triglycerides because of the low levels of insulin which puts the liver in a ketogenic mode.

There is a difference between low levels of insulin and absent insu-lin: in fasting, insulin, although low, is present in sufficient quanti-ties to prevent the unrestrained lipolysis and enhanced delivery of FFAs to the liver that characterizes the absence of insulin.

This is the difference between simple starvation and diabetic ketoacidosis (DKA); in the former, ketosis occurs but not ketoacidosis; in the latter, the total absence of insulin greatly enhances lipolysis which provides the substrate (FFAs) for unrestrained ketogenesis in liver with consequent ketoacidosis.

> Alcoholic ketoacidosis occurs in the setting of poor nutrient intake coupled with the very severe volume depletion that complicates serious alcohol abuse.

In this setting insulin secretion is suppressed by the sympathetic stimulation that accompanies alcohol-induced fluid losses (vomiting and diarrhea). SNS stimulation strongly inhibits insulin secretion by an α-adrenergic mechanism exerted on the pancreatic beta cells. In addition, the metabolism of ethanol increases the concentration of acetyl CoA in the liver by blocking entrance into the Krebs cycle and by blocking the oxidation of FFAs, thus enhancing ketone body formation.

> In distinction to DKA, alcoholic ketoacidosis is characteristically mild and responds readily to fluid resuscitation.

Other states of severe volume depletion may be associated with significant ketosis and ketoacidosis as well. Hyperemesis gravidarum and acute pancreatitis are common examples.

> In the presence of advanced renal insufficiency metformin may cause lactic acidosis.

Lactic acidosis was much more common with phenformin, the predecessor of metformin.

> The "delta gap" or the "delta-delta" calculation identifies a pre-existing acid–base disturbance in the presence of an acute anion gap acidosis.

By subtracting the normal anion gap (12) from the calculated anion gap (say 20) and adding the difference (8) to the measured bicarbonate concentration (say 22) it is possible to estimate the serum bicarbonate (30) at the onset of the anion gap acidosis, thereby identifying a pre-existing metabolic alkalosis.

Acidosis in Renal Disease

> Acidosis in the presence of renal disease is not associated with an increased anion gap until the renal disease is end stage.

Acidosis in renal disease is a consequence of either renal tubular dysfunction or the loss of sufficient renal mass to excrete the acid burden generated on a daily basis.

> In renal tubular acidosis (RTA) the urine cannot be acidified to the normal extent (pH below 5.3) because of either failure to reclaim bicarbonate from the glomerular filtrate (proximal RTA, type 2 RTA) or a defect in the excretion of hydrogen ions (distal RTA, type 1 RTA). The anion gap is normal. Type 4 RTA is aldosterone deficiency which prevents the distal acidification of the urine.

In the presence of severe reduction in GFR, below 25% of normal, plasma bicarbonate falls and chloride rises resulting in metabolic acidosis with a normal anion gap.

🔵 **The acidosis in advanced renal failure is caused by insufficient ammonium production to neutralize the daily acid burden.**

The urinary pH is appropriately low in renal failure and the ammonium production per functioning nephron is high, but there are insufficient nephrons to produce the adequate ammonium and the plasma pH falls. In more advanced renal failure the anion gap does increase as the retention of organic acids and phosphate increases and the chloride levels fall.

Metabolic Alkalosis

🔵 **Hypokalemic alkalosis, especially when severe and poorly responsive to potassium repletion, reflects mineralocorticoid excess.**

Hyperaldosteronism, either primary or secondary, is the usual but not the exclusive cause. These two forms of aldosterone excess are easily distinguished by plasma renin assay: suppressed in primary, elevated in secondary.

🔵 **Potassium chloride is the treatment of choice for metabolic alkalosis.**

Metabolic alkalosis usually occurs in the setting of chronic volume contraction and diminished renal perfusion, frequently a consequence of diuretic administration; the kidney, which is avidly reabsorbing sodium, must secrete hydrogen and potassium ions in exchange for sodium once chloride in the filtrate is completely reabsorbed. The result is inappropriately acidified urine in association with systemic alkalosis. The goal of treatment is to restore the ability of the kidney to sustain an alkaline diuresis by providing chloride, which permits sodium to be reabsorbed isoelectrically with the chloride. Since sodium is frequently inappropriate in the clinical setting, potassium chloride is the treatment of choice, since it also corrects the commonly associated potassium deficit.

Respiratory Alkalosis

🔵 **Respiratory alkalosis occurs acutely in the hyperventilation syndrome (psychogenic, panic attacks), salicylate intoxication, and sepsis, and chronically in hepatic encephalopathy.**

A positive Chvostek sign is a tip off to the diagnosis.

INTRINSIC RENAL DISEASE

Disease of the kidney may affect predominately the glomeruli or the interstitium. Both may result in chronic renal failure with small shrunken scarred kidneys. Statistically, glomerular diseases are more commonly associated with end stage renal failure.

Tubulointerstitial Disease

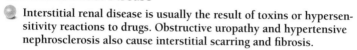 Interstitial renal disease is usually the result of toxins or hypersensitivity reactions to drugs. Obstructive uropathy and hypertensive nephrosclerosis also cause interstitial scarring and fibrosis.

Involvement initially spares the glomeruli, but eventually, scarring may involve the whole kidney and result in advanced renal failure. Tubular dysfunction with loss of renal concentrating ability may be prominent.

In distinction to glomerular diseases, proteinuria is absent or scant, and hematuria is not prominent in interstitial renal disease.

Drugs commonly involved include the penicillins, cephalosporins, NSAIDs, anticonvulsants, and analgesics. In the allergic form eosinophils may be present in the urine and increased in the peripheral blood.

In malignant hypertension proteinuria is nephrotic range and microscopic hematuria is common.

Fibrinoid arteriolar necrosis in the renal circulation is the cause.

Glomerulonephritis

Glomerulonephritis is the consequence of an immune attack on the kidney that results in damage and/or inflammation of the glomeruli. It may be primary or secondary, acute or chronic, focal or global; the glomerular epithelium, endothelium, or the basement membrane may be the primary target of the attack.

The autoimmune response is composed of different mechanisms in different disease entities. These include antibodies directed against the basement membrane of the glomerulus (membranous glomerulonephritis, Goodpasture syndrome); immune complex deposition from circulating or locally derived antigen–antibody interactions (IgA nephropathy, poststreptococcal glomerulonephritis (PSGN), lupus nephritis, serum sickness, subacute bacterial endocarditis); and so-called *pauci-immune* glomerulonephritis in which antigen–antibody complexes cannot be demonstrated (Wegener's, microscopic polyangiitis, ANCA-associated vasculitides).

Fixation and activation of complement contributes importantly to the glomerular injury in immune complex glomerulonephritis.

There is a corresponding decrease in circulating complement levels in renal diseases associated with immune complex deposition such as lupus nephritis and PSGN.

The clinical manifestations of glomerulonephritis are proteinuria and/or hematuria, hypertension, and in some cases edema and renal failure.

The red cell cast is virtually diagnostic of glomerular injury since it is formed in the renal tubules from protein and RBCs, thereby unequivocally establishing the provenance of the hematuria at the level of the injured glomerulus. Some non-inflammatory glomerular lesions produce only protein loss without hematuria.

🔘 **Renal biopsy is the usual means of identifying the various causes of glomerulonephritis, important since identification of the cause may have important therapeutic implications.**

Secondary glomerulonephritis occurs when renal involvement is part of a generalized disease such as SLE or Wegener's.

🔘 **PSGN is a prototypical immune complex glomerulopathy.**

A disease principally of children and less common today in the United States than previously, PSGN is still common worldwide and does occur in adults. The immunologic response to a group A beta-hemolytic streptococcal infection forms the immune complexes that fix complement with resultant glomerular injury.

🔘 **In distinction to acute rheumatic fever, which typically follows severe pharyngitis of any streptococcal serotype, PSGN is caused by specific nephritogenic strains, principally involving the skin.**

🔘 **Impetigo, or any impetiginized skin lesions with the appropriate nephritogenic strain of streptococci, can result in PSGN, indicating the importance of antibiotic treatment to eliminate the offending organism.**

The prognosis for full recovery of renal function in children is good, less so in adults.

🔘 **IGA nephropathy is the most common cause of primary glomerulone-phritis in adults.**

The immune deposits are autoantibodies to altered IgA. The glomerulonephritis is characterized by proteinuria and, frequently, gross hematuria. The glomerulonephritis may be self-limited or may progress to end stage renal disease.

🔘 **In children and young adults Henoch–Schönlein purpura is a gener-alized form of IgA deposition in which the skin (palpable purpura) and other organs are involved as well as the kidney.**

IgA deposition can be demonstrated in skin biopsy of the purpuric lesions.

Nephrotic Syndrome

Nephrotic syndrome refers to heavy proteinuria (in excess of 3 g/day) of any cause, and the complications pursuant to the loss of protein, of which there are many.

🔘 **The causes include diabetic nephropathy (Kimmelstiel–Wilson dis-ease also known as diabetic nodular glomerular sclerosis), various forms of primary and secondary glomerulonephritis, amyloidosis (AL and AA, primary and secondary amyloidosis respectively), and a large number of infections, drugs, toxins, and allergens.**

The clinical manifestations are edema, ascites, hyperlipidemia, and coagulopathies.

The pathogenesis of fluid accumulation reflects the decreased oncotic pressure of the plasma generated by the hypoalbuminemia and enhanced renal sodium reabsorption mediated at least in part by secondary aldosteronism. Protein synthesis in the liver is enhanced, including lipoprotein synthesis which, in conjunction with loss of lipoprotein lipase in the urine, results in hyperlipidemia. Loss of immunoglobulins results in increased susceptibility to infection, and loss of antithrombin III in the urine predisposes to venous thrombosis.

Treating the underlying cause, if possible, is frequently efficacious. Symptomatic treatment includes diuretics (loop plus spironolactone), statins, anticoagulation where appropriate, and aggressive surveillance for and treatment of infections.

Endocrinology and Metabolism

7

CHAPTER

DIABETES MELLITUS

Diabetic Complications

The introduction of routine insulin therapy prevented wasting and eventual death in ketoacidosis in patients with type 1 diabetes and uncontrolled glycosuria in type 2 patients. With increased survival the now well-recognized diabetic complications emerged and became the major long-term problem in patients with diabetes. For many years the debate raged as to whether "tight" control of the glucose lessened the complications. Studies were inconclusive because back then there was no tight control; what was compared was really awful control and just bad control. With the development of techniques for much better glucose control the issue has been pretty well settled.

 As a reasonable generalization the microvascular complications (retinopathy, nephropathy, and peripheral neuropathy) are markedly influenced by good blood glucose control, while the macrovascular complications (myocardial infarction, stroke, and peripheral vascular disease) are impacted much more by blood pressure control and much less by tight glucose control.

The pathogenesis of the micro- and macrovascular complications of diabetes are distinct: microvascular changes reflect the impact of high glucose concentrations on biochemical processes (advanced glycosylation end products, sorbitol accumulation, for example, as well as increased glomerular filtration); macrovascular complications represent accelerated atherosclerotic changes related to standard cardiovascular risk factors (blood pressure, lipids). The differences in pathogenetic mechanisms account for the differences in response to glucose lowering.

Microvascular complications are much more common in patients with type 1 diabetes than in patients with type 2; since type 2 is five times more common than type 1, however, there are more type 2 patients with microvascular complications in the population at large.

In type 1 diabetics the microvascular complications are related to the length of time that diabetes has been present; in type 2 patients microvascular complications may be present at the initial presentation.

This likely reflects the fact that the onset of type 1 diabetes is generally known with precision: a dramatic onset usually with ketoacidosis. In type 2 diabetes the onset is insidious rather than dramatic, and abnormal glucose metabolism is often present for years before diagnosis.

The cause of diabetes is always insulin deficiency but there is an important difference between type 1 and type 2: in type 1 the deficiency of insulin is absolute and complete; in type 2 the insulin deficiency is relative to the needs imposed by insulin resistance.

In type 2 the insulin levels are elevated compared with nondiabetic subjects but not elevated enough to lower the glucose levels to normal. Eventually, in many type 2 patients beta cell function slowly declines, necessitating treatment with insulin.

Diabetic Ketoacidosis

Diabetic ketoacidosis (DKA) develops in the complete absence of insulin, usually in the setting of type 1 diabetes mellitus (Table 7-1).

Under these circumstances lipolysis is totally unrestrained, free fatty acids are converted in the liver to ketone bodies (beta-hydroxybutyrate and oxaloacetate). Bedside testing with diluted serum and an Acetest tablet is sufficient to make the diagnosis in a patient with an anion gap.

Ketoacidosis never occurs in simple fasting since the amount of insulin available during a fast, although low, is not absent, and remains sufficient to prevent the unrestrained lipolysis characteristic of DKA.

TABLE 7.1 Diabetic Comas

Diabetic Ketoacidosis Endogenous Insulin Deficiency Absolute	Hyperosmolar Nonketotic Coma Endogenous Insulin Deficiency Relative
• Insulin therapy omitted	• Infection; glucocorticoid treatment
• Renal function normal	• Renal function impaired
• Blood glucose moderately elevated (300–400 mg/dL)	• Blood glucose markedly elevated (800–1,200 mg/dL)
• Urine ketones large	• Urine ketones absent to small
• Plasma ketoacids high	• Plasma ketoacids absent to low
• Anion gap acidosis severe	• Anion gap acidosis absent
• Volume depletion marked	• Volume depletion very severe
• Osmolality normal or high	• Osmolality high to very high

Simple fasting is associated with ketosis but the latter does not produce enough ketoacids to cause a metabolic acidosis. During fasting or starvation urine ketones are positive but serum ketones are absent or present in very low concentration.

 The commonest cause of DKA is failure to take insulin.

DKA frequently occurs in the setting of some (frequently mild) intercurrent illness in insulin-dependent diabetics; the patient, fearing that he or she will not be able to eat, omits insulin to avoid hypoglycemia. The intercurrent illness, however, increases insulin resistance and accentuates the need for insulin. More, not less, insulin is needed in these circumstances. This is an educational issue; patients should be instructed not to discontinue insulin when they become ill, but to follow "sick day rules" and contact their physician for instruction.

 DKA is associated with significant potassium depletion. The initial serum potassium level may be elevated (masking the deficit) because acidosis is associated with intracellular shifts of hydrogen ions and potassium.

The acidosis is buffered in part by cellular uptake of H^+ which is associated with potassium efflux into the extracellular space. As the acidosis diminishes during treatment the intracellular shifts are reversed and potassium levels fall. Potassium must be closely monitored and administered intravenously as the levels fall. A "normal" potassium level at presentation with acidosis necessitates potassium replacement from the outset.

 The EKG is a convenient way to assess potassium status at the bedside in DKA; initially high extracellular levels are reflected in high spiked T waves.

As the potassium level falls the T waves flatten indicating the need for replacement of potassium. Potassium levels should be measured hourly along with glucose, electrolytes, and the anion gap for as long as the ketoacidosis persists.

> The issues to be addressed in DKA are volume depletion, acidosis, hyperosmolality, hypoglycemia, and serum potassium levels.

Patients with DKA are severely volume depleted and dehydrated at presentation because of the osmotic diuresis produced by glycosuria, poor fluid intake, and occasionally, vomiting.

> The osmotic diuresis from uncontrolled glucosuria produces losses of water and salt (the urine osmolality during osmotic diuresis is about half normal saline, so more water than salt is lost).

This should be addressed by aggressive fluid resuscitation; normal saline can be given immediately, but a quick calculation of the osmolality (followed by a direct measurement in the laboratory) should be made and the infusate modified accordingly. Most patients will be hyperosmolar and require dilute fluids (half normal saline).

> A serum osmolality of 340 mOsm/kg or greater is an emergency that requires prompt treatment with hypotonic fluids.

Diffuse cerebral bleeding from brain shrinkage as the cortex pulls away from the meninges is the feared complication of hyperosmolar states.

> The primary treatment of the acidosis in DKA is to stop the production of ketoacids by administering insulin. Insulin stops the flux of free fatty acids (FFA) to the liver and promotes lipid, rather than ketoacid, synthesis.

Insulin should be administered by a bolus followed by continuous infusion. It is important to avoid hypoglycemia so when the plasma glucose falls into the range of 250 to 300 mg/dL, glucose (5%) should be added to the IV fluids. Unless the acidosis is very severe (pH below 7) and the blood pressure fails to respond to fluids, bicarbonate administration should be avoided.

There are several very good reasons to avoid bicarbonate in the treatment of DKA:

1. **It is sometimes associated with cerebral edema.** The mechanisms leading to this catastrophic complication are obscure but may involve oxygen delivery to the brain. In DKA red cell 2,3-diphoshoglycerate (2,3-DPG) is diminished due to the acidosis and perhaps to diabetes. 2,3-DPG is an important regulator of tissue oxygen delivery by changing the affinity of hemoglobin for oxygen: high levels of 2,3-DPG promote oxygen release, while low levels decrease oxygen delivery. In DKA the adverse effect of low 2,3-DPG is compensated by the independent effect of acidosis which decreases hemoglobin oxygen affinity, thereby promoting oxygen release. Bicarbonate administration, by rapidly changing the pH, leaves the adverse

effect of low 2,3-DPG unopposed and decreased oxygen delivery a possible result (see Fig 2.2). Whether this is responsible for the cerebral edema is not firmly established but the association of bicarbonate administration with the latter is well recognized.

2. **Bicarbonate induces a swift fall in serum potassium levels.** As described above acidosis induces a shift in potassium from the intracellular to the extracellular space so the initial level is frequently elevated masking severe potassium depletion; correcting the acidosis rapidly with bicarbonate leads to a rapid fall in potassium as cellular uptake of potassium increases; this shift may be associated with serious, sometimes fatal, arrhythmias. Accentuating hypokalemia during treatment is a serious problem.

3. **Endogenous bicarbonate is generated from glucose metabolism during successful treatment of DKA.** A metabolic alkalosis may develop if large amounts of bicarbonate have been administered in addition to insulin.

Hyperosmolar Nonketotic Coma

Hyperosmolar nonketotic coma (HONC) is a syndrome that usually occurs in noninsulin-dependent (usually type 2) diabetics (Table 7-1).

In distinction to type 1 patients those at risk for hyperosmolar coma are not devoid of insulin. Since the effects of insulin on inhibiting lipolysis are more sensitive than those stimulating muscle glucose uptake, these type 2 patients do not have unrestrained lipolysis and do not develop ketoacidosis. They suffer, rather, the effects of very high glucose levels. The associated volume depletion is usually severe and frequently associated with hyperosmolality.

Renal insufficiency is usually present allowing the glucose to rise to extremely high levels.

The osmotic diuresis results in water and salt loss with the greater deficit in water leading to the hyperosmolar state. Treatment is fluid resuscitation with hypotonic fluids and insulin. Glucose should be added to the fluids when the plasma glucose level reaches 300 mg/dL.

Intercurrent infections which increase insulin resistance and decrease fluid intake or treatment with glucocorticoids are common initiating events in HONC.

The mortality rate is high.

HYPOGLYCEMIA

Pathophysiology

Since the brain, for practical purposes, can utilize only glucose as an energy source hypoglycemia is completely analogous to hypoxia in its effects on neuronal function.

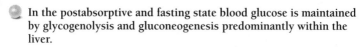 In the postabsorptive and fasting state blood glucose is maintained by glycogenolysis and gluconeogenesis predominantly within the liver.

The liver is almost completely depleted of glycogen after an overnight fast leaving gluconeogenesis as the prime defender of the blood glucose level in more prolonged fasts.

In advanced liver failure hypoglycemia may occur, but this is usually a preterminal event.

Spontaneous (endogenous) hypoglycemia occurs in either the fasting or the postprandial state. This is a clinically important distinction since the relationship of hypoglycemia to meals is an important clue to diagnosis (Table 7-2).

In both fasting and postprandial hypoglycemia the level of insulin is inappropriately high for the level of glucose.

Glucose Counterregulation

Hypoglycemia calls forth a counterregulatory hormonal response which increases the plasma glucose level. Glucagon and epinephrine are the principal counterregulatory hormones.

Increases in the secretion of these hormones, along with suppression of endogenous insulin release, raise the blood glucose level by stimulating hepatic glucose output (glycogenolysis and gluconeogenesis). Epinephrine contributes additionally by providing substrate (lactate) for gluconeogenesis from glycogenolysis in muscle, and by providing alternative substrate for nonneural tissues by stimulating lipolysis in adipose tissue.

The plasma glucose threshold for the initiation of the counterregulatory response is between 50 and 60 mg/dL.

Although cortisol and growth hormone (GH) are increased by hypoglycemia, neither of these hormones is involved in the acute counterregulatory response. Notwithstanding, the response of the pituitary to the intentional induction of hypoglycemia by intravenous insulin administration provides a convenient test of ACTH and GH reserve in the evaluation of pituitary function.

Symptoms of Hypoglycemia

Symptoms of hypoglycemia are of two types: adrenergic and neuroglycopenic.

Epinephrine release from the adrenal medulla as part of the counter regulatory response causes the adrenergic symptoms including palpitations and tremor along with the associated signs of tachycardia, widened pulse pressure, and increased systolic BP.

TABLE 7.2 Hypoglycemia

Fasting	Reactive (Postprandial)
Occurs after prolonged fast	Follows last meal within 5 hours
Neuroglycopenic symptoms predominate (seizures, coma)	Adrenergic symptoms predominate (sweating, palpitations)
Causes	**Causes**
Insulinoma (↑ c-peptide, proinsulin)	Exuberant insulin response (rapid gastric emptying); early type 2 diabetes (delayed insulin release)
Tumor hypoglycemia (insulin suppressed, ↑IGF 2)	
Exogenous insulin (c-peptide absent)	
Diagnosis	**Diagnosis**
Discordant insulin and glucose levels after fast	Discordant insulin and glucose levels during 5-hour glucose tolerance test

These epinephrine-induced symptoms form an early warning system for hypoglycemia. Sweating is prominent but not, as noted below, a consequence of epinephrine.

🔹 Impaired neuronal function is the manifestation of neuroglycopenia which includes confusion, dysarthria, impaired cognition, and in the extreme, seizures, coma, and even death.

🔹 Sweating, a very common manifestation of hypoglycemia, is cholinergically mediated eccrine sweating. It is due to the fall in temperature that occurs during hypoglycemia. Hypoglycemia is associated with mild hypothermia. Sweating dissipates heat to meet the new lower core temperature set point associated with hypoglycemia.

Patients may be drenched in sweat particularly during severe episodes. **It is a *faux pearl* that the sweating is adrenergically mediated.** Adrenergic sweating is apocrine in type and involves the axillary sweat glands and those about the upper lip. Hypoglycemic diaphoresis is generalized and involves the cholinergic sympathetic nerves.

🔹 Whipple's triad, the classic if self-evident criteria for the diagnosis of hypoglycemia, consists of: 1) compatible symptoms, 2) low measured glucose during the symptoms, and 3) relief with glucose administration.

The symptoms of hypoglycemia, particularly the adrenergic symptoms, are relatively nonspecific and mimic those caused by anxiety. A normal glucose during an episode categorically rules out hypoglycemia and thus the need for further evaluation. Most patients who believe that they have hypoglycemia do not fulfil Whipple's triad.

Causes of Hypoglycemia

◉ Drugs (insulin, sulfonylureas) are important causes of hypoglycemia.

◉ Exogenous insulin administration, by far the most common cause of hypoglycemia, is easily distinguished from endogenous hyperinsulinism by the absence of C peptide in the blood.

C peptide is the connecting piece of the insulin molecule that is cleaved during insulin synthesis and that is absent in commercial insulin preparations. It is released into the circulation along with insulin from the pancreatic beta cells.

◉ Insulin-induced hypoglycemia is usually a consequence of treatment for diabetes gone awry.

It is particularly common when the most intensive insulin regimens are employed.

◉ Insulin-induced hypoglycemia may also occur in suicide attempts or as a manifestation of factitious disease.

The latter should be suspected when hypoglycemia is noted in hospital workers or in the family of patients taking insulin.

◉ The physiologic side effects of epinephrine (tachycardia, palpitations, tremor), along with sympathetic cholinergic sweating, provide early warning signs of hypoglycemia.

When the epinephrine response is deficient, as in certain forms of autonomic failure, neuroglycopenia catches the patient unaware and may be associated with serious clinical manifestations such as seizures and coma.

◉ Hypoglycemia unawareness is a significant problem in long-term insulin-dependent diabetics and underlies the occurrence of repeated hypoglycemic episodes in these patients.

Failure of the glucagon response is common in long-standing insulin-dependent diabetics with absolute insulin deficiency. Insulin within the islets appears necessary to maintain glucagon responsiveness. To mount a counterregulatory response these diabetic patients are critically dependent on epinephrine; should autonomic failure develop the risk of repeated episodes of hypoglycemia is markedly increased.

◉ Fasting hypoglycemia occurs in the postabsorptive state well after the last meal. Insulinoma is the most common cause. Neuroglycopenic symptoms tend to dominate the clinical course.

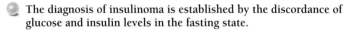 **The diagnosis of insulinoma is established by the discordance of glucose and insulin levels in the fasting state.**

This can be demonstrated by obtaining serial morning fasting plasma for glucose and insulin, or by a 72-hour fast. Measurements of C peptide level and proinsulin in plasma are also of value as these precursors of the mature insulin molecule may be elevated in patients with insulinoma.

Postprandial or "reactive" hypoglycemia occurs from 1 to 5 hours after a meal depending on the underlying disorder. The diagnosis can usually be established by a 5-hour glucose tolerance test with simultaneous measurements of insulin.

Higher than normal levels of insulin in response to the meal are presumed to be the cause, so that discordance between insulin and glucose levels occurs as the postprandial rise in glucose wanes while insulin is still present in sufficient quantities to lower the glucose into hypoglycemic ranges. Neuroglycopenic symptoms are very rare in reactive hypoglycemia, although they do occasionally occur. Hypoglycemia within an hour or two of a meal may occur in patients who have had gastric surgery (tachyalimentation) with rapid gastric emptying and a concomitant excessive rise in insulin. Hypoglycemia at 5 hours may be seen in early diabetes since the insulin response is delayed in these patients.

Fasting hypoglycemia may also be caused by nonbeta-cell tumors: tumor hypoglycemia.

Originally described with large, bulky, mesenchymal tumors the hypoglycemia was thought to result from glucose utilization by the tumor. This was never a very compelling explanation since hepatic glucose output was suppressed by the tumor and muscle glucose uptake was enhanced. Insulin production by the nonbeta-cell tumors was excluded as a cause, prompting a search for other humoral tumor products that might be responsible for these insulin-like effects.

Production of insulin-like growth factor 2 (IGF2) by the tumor is the cause of tumor hypoglycemia in the majority of cases. The hypoglycemia is frequently severe and may be the presenting manifestation of the tumor.

Incompletely processed IGF2 stimulates insulin receptors with resultant hypoglycemia. Insulin itself is suppressed. Many different types of tumor have been associated with this rare cause of hypoglycemia. Removing the tumor, wherever possible, is the treatment.

Alcoholic hypoglycemia occurs when ethanol is ingested in the starved state and maintenance of the plasma glucose is critically dependent on gluconeogenesis. The metabolism of the ethanol floods the liver with NADH, thereby blocking the synthesis of glucose from gluconeogenic precursors and disrupting the fasting equilibrium that maintained the plasma glucose by gluconeogenesis.

The typical picture of alcoholic hypoglycemia involves a serious alcoholic binge followed by a period of stupor. Fuel reserves are typically depleted by the preceding drunken spree and unconscious interval. On awakening alcohol consumption is resumed and the first drink initiates the biochemical cascade that blocks gluconeogenesis and hypoglycemia is the result.

MULTIPLE ENDOCRINE NEOPLASIA SYNDROMES

The multiple endocrine neoplasia (MEN) syndromes comprise three genetically and clinically distinct familial entities that result in adenomatous hyperplasia and malignant tumor formation in different endocrine organs (Table 7-3).

The clinical manifestations depend upon the pattern of glandular involvement and hormone secretion. All three have autosomal dominant inheritance with high penetration and variable expressivity. The genes involved have been identified and genetic screening is available for each syndrome.

MEN 1

MEN 1 involves the pancreas, the pituitary, and the parathyroid glands (the three Ps.).

TABLE 7.3 Multiple Endocrine Neoplasia (MEN) Syndromes

MEN-I	MEN-IIA	MEN-IIB
Wermer syndrome	Sipple syndrome	Mucosal neuroma syndrome
Mutation in tumor suppressor gene causing defect in transcription factor *menin*	*RET* proto-oncogene mutations with constitutive activation of receptor tyrosine kinase	
Hyperparathyroidism (adenomas) > 90% of affected	Hyperparathyroidism (adenomas) 25% of affected	Rare
Islet cell tumors 30–70% of affected	NO	NO
Pituitary tumors 50–65% of affected	NO	NO
Medullary carcinoma thyroid NO	>90% of affected	>90% of affected
Pheochromocytoma NO	50% of affected	60% of affected
Mucosal neuromas, Marfanoid habitus NO	NO	100% of affected

Any combination of tumors is possible; an affected individual with one of the tumors has a lifelong risk for the development of tumors in the other glands, necessitating lifelong screening. About 40% of affected persons develop tumors in all three glands. MEN 1 is caused by a mutation in a tumor suppressor gene that encodes a transcription factor called "menin."

- **Parathyroid tumors causing hypercalcemia are the most common manifestation of MEN 1 occurring in over 90% of affected individuals.**

Although asymptomatic hypercalcemia is most common, nephrolithiasis and nephrocalcinosis may occur. Diffuse parathyroid hyperplasia or multiple adenomas are more common than solitary adenomas, unlike the sporadic form of hyperparathyroidism in which a solitary adenoma predominates.

- **Pancreatic islet cell tumors occur in 60% to 70% of those affected with MEN 1; they may secrete insulin, gastrin, or vasoactive intestinal peptide (VIP) giving rise to syndromes based on hypersecretion of these hormones.**

Most tumors secrete pancreatic polypeptide as well, although the latter has no known clinical sequelae. Diffuse hyperplasia or multiple adenomas are the rule, and tumors may occur in the duodenal wall as well as in the pancreas.

- **Insulinomas originating from islet beta cells comprise about 40% of pancreatic tumors in MEN 1; they cause fasting hypoglycemia.**

Only a minority of patients with insulinoma, however, have the MEN 1 syndrome.

- **Gastrinomas originate from nonbeta-cell elements of the pancreas or the duodenal wall. They cause severe gastric acid overproduction (Zollinger–Ellison syndrome) which is associated with severe atypical peptic ulcer disease.**

About 50% of patients with gastrinomas have the MEN 1 syndrome.

- **Less common nonbeta-cell tumors secrete VIP (VIPomas) causing the syndrome of watery diarrhea, hypokalemia, and achlorhydria (WDHA, pancreatic cholera, Verner Morrison syndrome).**

Nonbeta-cell islet tumors in MEN 1 may also rarely secrete ACTH (causing Cushing's syndrome), calcitonin, and glucagon.

Carcinoid tumors of embryologic foregut origin giving rise to an atypical carcinoid syndrome is rarely associated as well.

- **Pituitary tumors in MEN 1 occur in less than 50% of affected patients; they may produce prolactin, GH, and very rarely, ACTH.**

Galactorrhea, infertility, impotence, acromegaly and, rarely, Cushing's disease may occur depending on the secretion products of the tumor.

MEN 2A

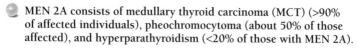 **MEN 2A consists of medullary thyroid carcinoma (MCT) (>90% of affected individuals), pheochromocytoma (about 50% of those affected), and hyperparathyroidism (<20% of those with MEN 2A).**

The genetic abnormality is well characterized (chromosome 10) and consists of mutations in the RET proto-oncogene that produces a constitutive activation in a receptor tyrosine kinase. All family members should be screened for this mutation.

Pheochromocytoma is the short-term immediate problem. Most kindreds have been identified by a symptomatic pheochromocytoma in the proband.

The pheochromocytomas in MEN 2A are always intra-adrenal, usually multicentric within the adrenal, preceded by adrenal medullary hyperplasia, frequently bilateral at presentation, and always epinephrine secreting.

Pheochromocytoma should be ruled out (measurement of urinary epinephrine and metanephrine) and, if present, addressed surgically before operation on the thyroid or parathyroids. If imaging reveals a unilateral tumor the involved adrenal should be removed and the patient followed for symptoms and biochemical evidence for involvement of the other adrenal. Bilateral tumors generally indicate the need for bilateral adrenalectomy.

MCT is the long-term problem since the tumor is frequently aggressive and fatal if untreated. It is preceded by C cell hyperplasia. Any affected individual should have a total thyroidectomy.

MCT is diagnosed by elevated calcitonin levels. Occasionally, the tumors produce other hormones such as ACTH which results in the ectopic ACTH syndrome. To reiterate, any family member with the trait should have a total thyroidectomy.

Parathyroid involvement in MEN 2A tends to be diffuse with hyperplasia or multiple adenomas.

The clinical manifestations result from hypercalcemia and the complications of hypercalcemia.

MEN 2B

MEN 2B results from a different mutation in the RET proto-oncogene; it consists of MCT, pheochromocytoma, and mucosal neuromas.

Hyperparathyroidism is not present. MCT is more aggressive than in MEN 2A.

The mucosal neuromas in MEN 2B present as glistening bumps on the eyelids and on hypertrophied lips.

Although the neuromas are presumably present since infancy, MEN 2B frequently escapes detection until early adult life when the syndrome presents with a thyroid mass or paroxysms related to the pheochromocytoma. Management of MCT and pheochromocytoma is the same as for MEN 2A.

⚫ **In MEN 2B marfanoid habitus is usually present and ganglioneuromas of the intestine may be associated with bowel motility problems.**

The causative mutation not infrequently arises *de novo* so the family history may be negative.

THYROID DISEASE

Thyroid Function Tests

⚫ **Thyroid stimulating hormone (TSH) is a reasonable screening test for thyroid disease, but if the clinical suspicion of thyroid disease in an individual patient is high, measurement of circulating thyroid hormones is required as well.**

When hyperthyroidism is under consideration a total triiodothyronine (T3) level should be obtained in addition to a free thyroxine (T4) level and TSH measurement.

⚫ **Normally, 75% to 80% of circulating T3 comes from peripheral conversion of T4; in endogenous hyperthyroidism much more T3 comes from the gland itself as the overactive gland is relatively iodine deficient.**

As a consequence in hyperthyroidism, particularly Graves' disease, the T3 level is usually elevated out of proportion to the level of T4.

⚫ **A normal T4 level and elevated T3 level has been referred to as "T3 toxicosis."**

⚫ **TSH levels are suppressed in all forms of thyrotoxicosis except in the very rare situation of a pituitary adenoma secreting TSH.**

⚫ **Radioactive iodine (RAI) uptake and scan should be obtained in virtually all cases of hyperthyroidism in order to establish the underlying cause.**

With the exception of the situations described below hyperthyroidism is associated with increased RAI. In Graves' disease the uptake is diffuse; with a toxic adenoma the uptake is localized to the nodule and suppressed in the remainder of the gland; and in toxic multinodular goiter there are areas of increased uptake interspersed with areas of decreased uptake.

⚫ **Hyperthyroidism with a low RAI has a limited and specific differential diagnosis: iodine excess; subacute and postpartum thyroiditis; factitious thyrotoxicosis; and struma ovarii (Table 7-4).**

Expansion of the endogenous iodine pool occurs with therapeutic doses of sodium iodide or the antiarrhythmic agent amiodarone; the RAI administered

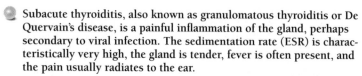

TABLE 7.4 Hyperthyroidism with a Low RAI Uptake

- Iodide excess (inorganic I or I-radiocontrast media)
- Subacute thyroiditis
- Lymphocytic or postpartum thyroiditis
- Factitious hyperthyroidism
- Struma ovarii

to assess uptake is diluted in the greatly expanded pool giving a falsely low calculated uptake of the tracer.

Subacute thyroiditis, also known as granulomatous thyroiditis or De Quervain's disease, is a painful inflammation of the gland, perhaps secondary to viral infection. The sedimentation rate (ESR) is characteristically very high, the gland is tender, fever is often present, and the pain usually radiates to the ear.

The thyroid hormone response is characteristically biphasic; increased release of preformed hormone at the outset followed by a hypothyroid phase after a few weeks with return to normal after a few months. Antithyroid drugs are of no use since thyroid hormone synthesis is not increased. Beta blockers may be used for symptomatic relief of hyperthyroid symptoms along with anti-inflammatories.

Postpartum thyroiditis is painless and occurs 3 to 6 months postpartum. A hyperthyroid phase is succeeded by a period of hypothyroidism followed by recovery in most cases.

There is no role for antithyroid drugs.

Surreptitious ingestion of thyroid hormone causes factitious hyperthyroidism, a psychiatric illness most common in health care workers. Goiter is absent.

Struma ovarii is a very rare disease caused by aberrant thyroid tissue in an ovarian teratoma. RAI is increased over the ovaries but suppressed in the neck.

Hyperthyroidism

Graves' disease, the most common form of hyperthyroidism, is an autoimmune disease in which thyroid-stimulating immunoglobulins (TSIs) interact positively with the thyroid TSH receptor resulting in diffuse stimulation of the gland.

A bruit over the thyroid, reflecting increased blood flow, is virtually diagnostic of Graves' disease.

Graves' disease is much more common in women than in men. The diagnosis can be confirmed by measuring TSI in the blood.

● Although the cause of Graves' disease is immunologic, the disease may be precipitated by a severe emotional shock.

Among the stressful situations known to initiate hyperthyroidism in Graves' patients are an automobile accident (being hit in the rear), a fire in the house, or a death in the family. Perhaps activation of the sympathetic nervous system is involved since the thyroid follicular epithelium is innervated and SNS stimulation is known to increase thyroid hormone release.

● Graves' ophthalmopathy is due to swelling and infiltration of the orbital contents, including the extraocular muscles, with fibrosis, fat, and inflammatory cells. The resulting proptosis may be unilateral or bilateral.

In addition to lid lag, widened palpebral fissure, and stare, which may occur in all forms of hyperthyroidism, true proptosis occurs only in Graves' disease.

● The physical findings in Graves' ophthalmopathy include, in addition to proptosis, diplopia most marked on upward outward gaze, conjunctival injection, and in severe cases retinal hemorrhages and papilledema that threaten vision.

Severe ophthalmopathy is much more common in current smokers.

● Graves' disease is the most common cause of unilateral exophthalmos in adults.

CT scan is useful in ruling out tumor invasion of the orbit, pseudotumor oculi, or cavernous sinus thrombosis.

● A bruit over the orbit occurs in the rare case of unilateral exophthalmos secondary to a carotid cavernous sinus fistula.

● Many of the clinical findings in hyperthyroidism reflect the increase in metabolic rate induced by thyroid hormone excess. Some of the findings reflect heightened SNS responses which are potentiated by thyroid hormone excess.

The weight loss, sweating, and heat intolerance are obvious examples, but the cardiovascular symptoms reflect the increase in metabolic rate as well, since any increase in oxygen consumption must be accompanied by an increase in cardiac output. Thus pulse rate and pulse pressure are elevated, the latter being a good surrogate indicator of cardiac output. The peripheral resistance and mean BP are reduced. **It is a *faux pearl* that hyperthyroidism is associated with hypertension.**

Proximal muscle weakness also reflects the catabolic state. Widened palpebral fissure, tremor, and rapid reflex return reflect, in part, enhanced SNS responses in the presence of thyroid hormone excess and are ameliorated by beta blockade.

"Apathetic" hyperthyroidism is sometimes encountered in elderly patients who develop thyrotoxicosis from a multinodular goiter or Graves' disease. The usual hyperkinetic signs are absent and the clinical picture is dominated by weight loss and muscle atrophy.

In those patients with Graves' disease goiter may be absent or difficult to appreciate. Atrial fibrillation and heart failure may be present. The usual treatment is RAI ablation and the improvement is frequently astonishing to the patient and the patient's relatives.

Hypothyroidism

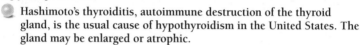 Hashimoto's thyroiditis, autoimmune destruction of the thyroid gland, is the usual cause of hypothyroidism in the United States. The gland may be enlarged or atrophic.

Hashimoto's thyroiditis is the other end of the spectrum of autoimmune thyroid disease; in distinction to Graves' disease where TSI stimulate the thyroid, the autoimmune process in Hashimoto's destroys the gland. Antibodies to thyroid peroxidase (TPO) are useful diagnostically but the actual autoimmune destruction is principally due to lymphocytic infiltration.

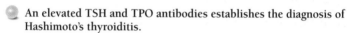 An elevated TSH and TPO antibodies establishes the diagnosis of Hashimoto's thyroiditis.

Other causes of hypothyroidism include iodine deficiency (associated with goiter) in those inland parts of the world where iodine deficiency is endemic and post-RAI ablation in the treatment of hyperthyroidism.

As noted above there is also a hypothyroid phase in the evolution of subacute thyroiditis and postpartum thyroiditis.

The skin in hypothyroidism is usually dry and scaly resembling icthyosis; it may also take on a yellowish hue due to hypercarotenemia, particularly noticeable on the palms, and secondary to decreased metabolism of beta-carotene. Hypothermia and somnolence occur in severe cases particularly in the winter months.

Although most processes are slowed down in hypothyroidism, the SNS is stimulated, perhaps as compensation for the decrease in thermogenesis and the reduced cardiac output. The blood pressure is increased in hypothyroidism and the peripheral resistance is increased. Treatment reverses these manifestations.

The "sick euthyroid" syndrome is common in very ill or starving patients. It is frequently seen in intensive care units. The T3 level is low due to impaired conversion of T4 to T3.

This syndrome is not a disease of the thyroid and needs no specific treatment. This may be a part of a conservative mechanism to diminish energy expenditure in the face of a catabolic state induced by severe illness or injury.

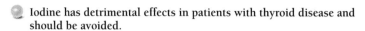 **Iodine has detrimental effects in patients with thyroid disease and should be avoided.**

In iodine deficiency goiter the provision of excess iodine to a gland that has enlarged in the effort to extract every bit of iodine from a deficient diet results in florid hyperthyroidism (the Jod-Basedow effect). The treatment of iodine deficient goiter is thyroxine (not iodine). The same phenomenon applies in multinodular goiter, but in less dramatic form. The iodine in x-ray contrast media is often sufficient to produce hyperthyroidism. In patients with Hashimoto's thyroiditis hypothyroidism may result from large doses of iodine because the gland does not escape from the suppressive effect of iodine (the Wolff–Chaikoff effect) the way a normal gland does.

CALCIUM

Calcium measurement without a corresponding albumin level is uninterpretable and therefore useless. A 1 g/dL fall in albumin is associated with a 1 mg /dL fall in total calcium. Ionized calcium, not routinely measured, is tightly controlled by parathyroid hormone.

Hypercalcemia

It is a cliché, but often correct, that hypercalcemia noted in outpatients is hyperparathyroidism, while hypercalcemia discovered in hospitalized patients is secondary to malignancy.

This is especially true when hypercalcemia is noted incidentally on multiphasic screening panels. The diagnosis is settled by measurement of parathyroid hormone levels, although a measurement of 24-hour urine calcium should be obtained to rule out familial hypocalciuric hypercalcemia (FHH) especially if there is a family history of hypercalcemia.

In FHH mild hypercalcemia is associated with very low 24-hour urinary calcium excretion due to faulty sensing of calcium by the parathyroid glands and the kidneys.

This is a benign familial disorder (autosomal dominant inheritance) which requires no treatment.

Hypercalcemia of malignancy is a paraneoplastic syndrome associated with many different types of neoplastic disease.

In most, but not all cases, routine age-appropriate clinical evaluation will reveal the tumor responsible. The mechanisms of tumor hypercalcemia have been well worked out and differ between solid and liquid (hematologic) malignancies.

Hypercalcemia caused by solid tumors has a humoral basis (humoral hypercalcemia of malignancy) (HHM): production of parathyroid hormone-related protein (PTHrP) which activates the parathyroid hormone receptor.

In the HHM syndrome bony metastases may be present or absent. The hypercalcemia depends on the effects of PTHrP rather than on direct dissolution of skeletal bone by the tumor. Although many tumors produce PTHrP squamous cell lung cancer and renal cell carcinoma are most commonly associated with the HHM syndrome. Since PTHrP is absent from the plasma in normal individuals, the diagnosis of HHM is made from measurement of PTHrP in the presence of hypercalcemia.

When metastases are extensive bony dissolution by tumor may contribute to hypercalcemia as well.

🔹 **Hematologic malignancies, of which multiple myeloma is the prototype, cause the direct dissolution of bone by the action of locally produced cytokines (osteoclast activating factors) with attendant hypercalcemia.**

Since the lesions produced by these factors are purely lytic alkaline phosphatase levels and conventional bone scans are normal since these tests measure osteoblastic activity. Solid tumor metastases to bone, even those that appear purely lytic by conventional radiography, have a small rim of osteoblastic activity around them and it is this osteoblastic reaction that elevates the alkaline phosphatase and shows up on bone scans.

🔹 **Hypervitaminosis D and A are also causes of hypercalcemia.**

Supplements sold in health food stores may have unpredictable amounts of vitamins and food faddists may take these in large quantities.

🔹 **Hypervitaminosis A is also associated with increased intracranial pressure.**

Hypocalcemia

The important and well known causes of hypocalcemia include hypoparathyroidism (postsurgical or autoimmune), vitamin D deficiency, chronic renal failure (failure to produce 1,25-dihydroxy D), and hyperphosphatemia (precipitation of calcium).

🔹 **Rare, but potentially important, causes of hypocalcemia include acute pancreatitis (fat necrosis with saponification – the formation of calcium soaps which precipitate), and osteoblastic metastases when extensive (prostate cancer).**

🔹 **Hypomagnesemia is associated with hypocalcemia and hypophosphatemia and should be suspected when both calcium and phosphate are low.**

Most common in alcoholics and as a consequence of long-term diuretic usage, magnesium repletion is essential to restore serum calcium levels to normal.

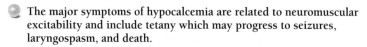 The major symptoms of hypocalcemia are related to neuromuscular excitability and include tetany which may progress to seizures, laryngospasm, and death.

Latent tetany may be elicited by Chvostek and/or Trousseau sign: facial twitch on tapping the facial nerve over the parotid gland and carpopedal spasm when a blood pressure cuff is inflated above the systolic pressure.

Hyperventilation is often associated with latent tetany and a normal measured calcium level since respiratory alkalosis decreases ionized calcium by increasing calcium binding to serum proteins.

Hypoparathyroidism is associated with basal ganglia calcification which may cause extrapyramidal neurologic symptoms.

Hypophosphatemia

A not uncommon finding in hospitalized patients, hypophosphatemia has many causes, and, depending on the circumstances, several consequences which may be significant. The common causes of hypophosphatemia include increased cellular phosphate uptake, increased urinary phosphate excretion, and decreased GI phosphate absorption.

Refeeding after a period of starvation, or during the treatment of uncontrolled diabetes with insulin, a marked intracellular uptake of phosphate occurs. The intracellular phosphate is utilized in cellular glucose metabolism and glycogen synthesis.

In the recovery phase of diabetic ketoacidosis the fall in phosphate may be quite remarkable since the enhanced cellular uptake is superimposed on an underlying phosphate deficiency from urinary losses in the osmotic diuresis and diminished phosphate intake that occur in the run up to DKA.

Respiratory alkalosis is a common cause of hypophosphatemia since the increased alkaline environment in the cells stimulates glycolysis and the utilization of phosphate.

This mechanism contributes to the hypophosphatemia that occurs in alcoholics and cirrhotics, and is the cause of the hypophosphatemia in then hyperventilation syndrome. In the latter case a positive Chvostek sign secures the diagnosis.

Excessive phosphaturia occurs in hyperparathyroidism (primary or secondary), vitamin D deficiency or resistance, renal phosphate wasting disorders, and oncogenic osteomalacia.

PTH directly stimulates phosphate excretion. In vitamin D deficiency secondary hyperparathyroidism occurs along with impairment in phosphate absorption from the gut. Renal phosphate wasting may be part of a generalized renal tubular disease in which many essential substances are lost in the urine (Fanconi's syndrome); rickets is a common consequence.

Phosphate wasting without the loss of other substrates or minerals occurs in X-linked vitamin D resistant rickets and oncogenic osteo-malacia. In both cases the phosphaturic protein fibroblast growth factor (FGF) 23 is responsible.

In the inherited X-linked dominant syndrome a mutant form of FGF 23 is resistant to normal breakdown so that the higher levels stimulate phosphate excretion. In oncogenic osteomalacia FGF 23 is produced as a paraneoplastic hormone and the increased levels drive phosphate excretion.

The tumors secreting FGF 23 tend to be small and mesenchymal, not malignant, sometimes located in bone, and characteristically difficult to localize. Tumor removal results in cure of the phosphaturia.

 The clinical manifestations of hypophosphatemia depend upon the severity and the presence or absence of total body phosphate depletion. Metabolic encephalopathy and muscle weakness are severe manifestations. Depletion of RBC 2,3-DPG may impair oxygen delivery to tissues by shifting the hemoglobin oxygen dissociation curve to the right (Fig. 2-2).

Severe cases, particularly in alcoholics, may lead to rhabdomyolysis. In the intensive care unit hypophosphatemia may antagonize weaning patients from their ventilatory support.

POLYURIA

Polyuria is a common presenting complaint with an extensive differential diagnosis. The first question to be answered is whether nocturia is present and the next is whether the frequent voiding is large volume or small.

 Nocturia validates the complaint of excessive urination. Frequent small voiding suggests a urinary tract problem (cystitis, prostatism); large volume raises the possibility a renal or endocrine cause.

Loss of concentrating capacity by the kidney may reflect renal disease or the gradual loss of concentrating ability with aging.

 Endocrine causes of polyuria include hypercalcemia and hypokalemia (which impair renal concentrating ability), and diabetes mellitus (osmotic diuresis from glucosuria) as well as diabetes insipidus (DI) (deficiency of antidiuretic hormone [ADH]).

The Posterior Pituitary Gland (Diabetes Insipidus [DI])

One of the central problems in evaluating polyuria and polydipsia is ruling out DI since diabetes mellitus is excluded by the absence of weight loss and dipstick urine analysis for glucose.

 Central DI is caused by failure of the hypothalamus and posterior pituitary to produce ADH in sufficient quantities to reabsorb free water at the level of the renal distal tubule and collecting duct. The leading cause is "idiopathic" but secondary causes need to be ruled out.

ADH, also known synonymously as arginine vasopressin (AVP), is required to reabsorb water from the distal nephron; in the absence of ADH the distal tubule and medullary collecting duct are impermeable to water.

ADH is made in neurons of the supraoptic and periventricular nuclei of the hypothalamus; the axons of these neurons traverse the pituitary stalk and form the posterior pituitary or neurohypophysis. Why ADH production fails suddenly in idiopathic DI is unknown.

- **The onset of idiopathic central DI is characteristically sudden. Patients can frequently recall the precise moment at which the DI symptoms began ("I was sitting on my porch when…").**

- **Patients with DI crave ice water, in distinction to other drinks, and consume prodigious amounts to keep up with urinary water losses.**

The main differential diagnosis is with psychogenic polydipsia, the voluntary ingestion of large amounts of liquids, often occurring in association with significant psychiatric disease. The issue can be satisfactorily resolved by a water deprivation test. The latter must be carefully supervised since patients with DI fail to reduce urine output risking severe dehydration. Patients with psychogenic polydipsia will concentrate their urine above plasma, although washout of the medullary gradient, which drives back diffusion of water in the presence of ADH, may limit the concentrating ability of the psychogenic drinkers.

- **Central DI is easily distinguished from nephrogenic DI by the response to exogenous ADH.**

At the end of the water deprivation test the administration of ADH causes a sharp fall in urine output and corresponding increase in urine concentration in patients with central DI. Patients with nephrogenic DI, in which the kidneys cannot respond normally to ADH, have a subnormal response to the exogenous hormone.

- **ADH has a vanishingly short half-life in plasma. The synthetic congener DDAVP (desmopressin) is used as therapy and in testing.**

The development of DDAVP was a major therapeutic advance in the treatment of DI since it controls polyuria for long periods of time. DDAVP was one of the first "designer" drugs since it was specifically designed to avoid the rapid metabolism and the pressor effects of the natural AVP.

- **Patients with DI do not suffer volume depletion nor hypernatremia as long as their thirst mechanism is intact. The serum sodium level does not distinguish between psychogenic polydipsia and DI.**

With an intact thirst mechanism DI patients drink enough to keep up with the urinary water losses. When unconscious for any reason careful monitoring of intake and output and as well as frequent measurement of the serum sodium level is required.

● Gestational DI is a transient form of DI that occurs during pregnancy, usually in the third trimester. It is due to increased metabolism of endogenous AVP by a placental amino peptidase.

This syndrome, which remits shortly (days to weeks) after delivery, may be associated with antecedent subclinical central DI. DDAVP is not affected and is useful as treatment.

● Secondary central DI results from destruction of the posterior pituitary, pituitary stalk and infundibulum of the hypothalamus by tumor, infiltrative diseases, pituitary surgery, and head trauma.

Tumors of the anterior pituitary are not usually associated with DI unless they are very large and involve the pituitary stalk. There is sufficient ADH reserve in the hypothalamic neurohypophyseal tracts to prevent the development of full blown DI. Craniopharyngiomas, on the other hand, since they frequently develop in the region of the pituitary stalk, often present with DI.

● Metastatic tumor deposits in the pituitary or at the base of the skull may also cause DI; breast is the classic metastatic carcinoma associated with DI but carcinoma of the lung is also a common cause.

Infiltrative diseases such sarcoidosis and histiocytosis X (Hand–Schüller–Christian disease, eosinophilic granuloma) may cause central DI as well.

● Spontaneous pneumothorax in a patient with DI is always caused by eosinophilic granuloma.

ANTERIOR PITUITARY

Prolactin

High levels of prolactin are associated with hypogonadism in men and women. Galactorrhea occurs in women if the breast has had the appropriate endocrine priming.

● Hyperprolactinemia may be caused by tumor (prolactinoma), lesions that disrupt the pituitary stalk, or drugs.

The highest circulating prolactin levels (over 100 μg/L) are caused by adenomas of the anterior pituitary. Many drugs produce modest prolactin elevations but neuroleptic agents that antagonize dopamine (DA) are the most common culprits.

● Hypothyroidism may also be associated with elevations in prolactin that fall with appropriate treatment.

Prolactin is the only anterior pituitary hormone that is under tonic inhibition. DA, elaborated in hypothalamic regulatory neurons, inhibits the release of prolactin from the lactotropes of the anterior pituitary.

- **Lesions affecting the pituitary stalk disrupt the tonic inhibition imposed by DA resulting in enhanced secretion of prolactin.**

Drugs that block the action of DA result in hyperprolactinemia. Dopaminergic agonists are useful in treating pituitary adenomas secreting prolactin.

- **Kallmann syndrome refers to a specific subset of patients with hypogonadotropic hypogonadism and anosmia (absent sense of smell).**

In this syndrome luteinizing hormone (LH) and follicle stimulating hormone (FSH) are deficient due to a failure of the hypothalamus to produce gonadotropic-releasing hormone, which normally regulates the secretion of LH and FSH. Although it occurs in males and females it has a strong male predominance. The anosmia reflects poor development of the olfactory bulb. Hypogonadotropic hypogonadism also occurs with a normal sense of smell, but Kallmann syndrome refers specifically to the form with anosmia.

- **The presence of anosmia can be elicited by the question: have you ever smelled bacon cooking? (Almost everybody has!)**

The disease is characterized by the combination of low gonadal hormones with low LH and FSH levels. Puberty is delayed and incomplete, testes are very small, secondary sex characteristics are absent or poorly developed, and in females presentation is frequently with primary amenorrhea.

Growth Hormone

- **Acromegaly is caused by GH-secreting tumors that develop in adulthood after fusion of the epiphyses of the long bones. Before epiphyseal closure GH excess causes gigantism, also known as giantism.**

Most effects of GH are mediated by IGF 1, elaborated principally in the liver under the influence of GH. Measurement of IGF 1 (previously called somatomedin-C) in plasma is useful as a diagnostic test for GH excess.

- **In adults growth of the flat bones of the face causes broadening of the nose and brow, prognathism, and increased spacing between the teeth. The latter is the most useful and specific sign of acromegaly.**

Is it just a face with a broad nose and coarsened features or is it acromegaly? Widely spaced teeth make it acromegaly.

Osteoarthritis is common in GH excess because of growth of the ends of the long bones distorts the joint surfaces. Acral overgrowth also results in an increase in glove and shoe size. Heel pad thickness is increased.

There is an increased incidence of colon polyps and cancer in patients with GH excess presumably due to the stimulatory effects of IGF 1 on cell growth.

Cardiovascular disease (the usual cause of death) and diabetes mellitus are also more common in patients with acromegaly.

Pituitary Infarction

"Pituitary apoplexy" refers to the acute catastrophic hemorrhagic infarction of the pituitary with swelling of the intrasellar contents and the attendant hormonal and neurologic consequences.

The onset is commonly heralded by retro-orbital headache and ophthalmoplegia, followed by coma in severe cases. The usual cause is hemorrhage into a pituitary tumor necessitating neurosurgical evacuation of the hematoma in all but the mildest cases. The ophthalmoplegia reflects pressure on the cavernous sinuses, which form the lateral walls of the sella turcica, and consequent pressure on the third, fourth, and sixth cranial nerves which traverse these sinuses.

During pregnancy the pituitary normally swells and the blood flow increases rendering the gland, which sits in a rigid structure (the sella turcica), prone to infarction in the face of obstetrical emergency, particularly brisk hemorrhage (Sheehan's syndrome).

In distinction to apoplexy the infarction that follows is usually silent but leads, in the ensuing weeks to years, to panhypopituitarism.

Failure of lactation is usually the first manifestation of postpartum pituitary failure.

Amenorrhea followed by thyroid and adrenal deficiency complete the clinical picture. Imaging reveals an "empty sella."

Cerebrospinal Fluid (CSF) Rhinorrhea

Copious, clear, nonsticky fluid from the nose in the absence of infection or allergy, should raise the suspicion of a CSF leak, which may be caused by aggressive pituitary tumors, trauma, postsurgical manipulation in the region of the sell turcica, and increased intracranial pressure.

The time-honored bedside diagnostic test is the demonstration of a positive test for glucose on a glucose oxidase dip-stick.

Alas, this simple test has fallen into disfavor because contamination with blood may give false-positive results and in situations in which CSF glucose is low, false negatives. The CSF protein moiety beta-2 transferrin (not found in blood) is recommended as more specific, but in the right clinical circumstance of copious clear fluid the glucose dipstick is quite useful and the result immediately available.

ADRENAL CORTEX

Adrenal Function Testing

Hypofunction of the adrenal cortex is diagnosed by the failure of the gland to respond to stimulation with ACTH; overactivity of the adrenal cortex is diagnosed by the failure of the gland to suppress steroid output in response to glucocorticoid administration. Synthetic ACTH is used in the stimulation tests; the potent synthetic steroid dexamethasone is used in the suppression tests.

Synthetic ACTH (0.25 mg), consisting of the first 24 amino acid residues of the intact ACTH polypeptide (cosyntropin), is utilized in the stimulation test. Blood samples are obtained at 0, 30, and 60 minutes; the test may be performed at any time of the day. Criteria for a normal response include an increment of 7 µg/dL and an achieved value of at least 18 µg/dL. Although this test does not measure pituitary ACTH reserve, a normal response is usually taken to mean that the axis will support an adequate adrenal cortical response to severe illness or surgery, an assumption borne out by clinical experience.

Adrenal Insufficiency

The major causes of primary adrenal insufficiency (Addison disease) are destruction of the gland by an autoimmune process, by infection, by hemorrhage, or by metastatic cancer. In primary adrenal insufficiency both mineralocorticoid and glucocorticoid functions are lost.

Idiopathic Addison disease, the most common form of primary adrenal insufficiency, is the consequence of an immunologic attack by autoantibodies and T cells. In times past tuberculosis was the most common cause. Other infections can involve the adrenals as well, particularly granulomatous diseases and especially in patients with AIDS.

Although the adrenals are common sites of metastatic deposits, rarely do tumor metastases result in adrenal insufficiency since most of the adrenal needs to be destroyed or replaced before clinical manifestations of insufficiency appear.

The lung is the most common primary tumor that metastases to the adrenals and adenocarcinomas are the most common cell type.

Bilateral adrenal hemorrhage is rare but usually causes acute (followed by chronic) adrenal insufficiency. Adrenal hemorrhage most frequently occurs in patients who are anticoagulated or have an underlying coagulopathy.

Many of these events occur during surgical procedures or stressful illnesses.

The usual presentation of adrenal hemorrhage is with shock and flank or back pain. Imaging shows bilateral adrenal masses.

Prompt resuscitation with stress dose steroids and saline is lifesaving.

The clinical findings in chronic primary adrenal insufficiency include weight loss, fatigue, muscle weakness, nausea and vomiting, abdominal pain, low blood pressure, and hyperpigmentation.

Hyperkalemia (no aldosterone), hyponatremia (volume depletion), eosinophilia (low cortisol), narrow heart on chest x-ray (low volume), and high calcium level are frequently noted. The latter is in bound form and therefore exerts no physiologic effects. The ACTH level is elevated, useful diagnostically, and responsible for the hyperpigmentation.

 In adrenal insufficiency secondary to pituitary failure aldosterone is not affected so volume depletion is absent as is hyperpigmentation since ACTH levels are low.

Hyponatremia in secondary adrenal insufficiency is dilutional and reflects glucocorticoid deficiency; in the absence of a permissive amount of cortisol the distal renal tubule and collecting duct are permeable to water even in the absence of ADH.

Potassium is normal in secondary adrenal insufficiency. Mineralocorticoid replacement is not required in secondary adrenal insufficiency in distinction to the primary form which requires the synthetic mineralocorticoid fludrocortisone in addition to cortisol or prednisone.

 Adrenal insufficiency may be part of a familial autoimmune polyglandular failure constellation (Schmidt's syndrome) that includes the pituitary, the ovaries, the thyroid, and the endocrine pancreas.

Also known as polyglandular autoimmune syndrome type 2 (PAS 2), the inheritance is complex and not fully understood. PAS 1 is a disease of childhood and includes mucocutaneous candidiasis and hypoparathyroidism. Other autoimmune diseases associated with Schmidt syndrome include vitiligo, alopecia, premature graying of the hair, myasthenia gravis, and pernicious anemia.

Adrenal Suppression

 Clinically significant adrenal suppression from exogenous glucocorticoid administration is the most common form of adrenal insufficiency encountered clinically; suppression may be assumed to be present if the patient has been on a suppressive dose of prednisone (over 20 mg/day or equivalent of other glucocorticoid) for over 14 days. Suppressed adrenal function should be inferred for 1 year after the glucocorticoid has been stopped.

Although opinion varies it is wise to give stress dose steroids if the patient has had a suppressive dose of glucocorticoid for over 2 weeks during the past year. With less than 14 days of therapy it is generally safe to assume that the patient is not suppressed. After 1 year without steroids it is generally safe to assume that the patient is no longer suppressed.

🔵 **Stress dose steroids should mirror the maximum cortisol output achieved under naturally occurring conditions.**

Although maximal steroid output is the equivalent of 300 mg of hydrocortisone per day, a replacement dose of about 200 to 250 mg/day of cortisol IV (or its equivalent) in the face of severe illness or surgery is usually sufficient.

🔵 **Aldosterone secretion is regulated by angiotensin II and potassium and not by ACTH. In cases of adrenal suppression and pituitary insufficiency, therefore, it is not necessary to replace mineralocorticoids.**

Although plasma aldosterone levels increase acutely in response to ACTH the increase is not sustained and aldosterone regulation is known to be normal in the absence of ACTH.

Adrenocortical Excess

🔵 Cushing's syndrome is the general term for glucocorticoid excess; Cushing's disease refers to hypercortisolism secondary to excessive secretion of ACTH from the pituitary gland, usually from a microadenoma of the pituitary corticotrophs (Table 7-5).

TABLE 7.5 Cushing Syndrome

Cause	ACTH Level	Diagnosis	Clinical Features
Pituitary microadenoma	↑	Fails to suppress on low-dose dex; suppresses on high-dose dex	Classic stigmata: moon face, buffalo hump; broad purple striae; hypertension
Ectopic ACTH syndrome	↑↑	Fails to suppress on high-dose dex	Hypokalemic alkalosis; hyperpigmentation; hypertension; weakness; diabetes
Adrenal adenoma	↓↓	Fails to suppress on high-dose dex; imaging	Classic stigmata
Adrenal carcinoma	↓↓	Fails to suppress on high-dose dex; ↑ adrenal androgens; imaging	Large mass; classic stigmata + androgenic effects
Exogenous glucocorticoids	↓↓	Fails cosyntropin stimulation test	Classic stigmata; weakness; steroid psychosis

Cushing's disease is the most common cause of endogenous cortisol excess accounting for more than two-thirds of the cases. The iatrogenic syndrome, an undesirable consequence of glucocorticoid use as an anti-inflammatory or immunosuppressive agent, is the most common cause overall.

● The low-dose dexamethasone test (0.5 mg q6h for 2 days) is used to establish a diagnosis Cushing's syndrome; the high-dose dexamethasone test (2.0 mg q6h for 2 days) is used to distinguish Cushing's disease from the other forms of Cushing's syndrome. A positive response is suppression of 24-hour urinary-free cortisol and plasma cortisol to very low levels.

● The plasma cortisol level following an overnight dose of dexamethasone is a good screening test; after 1 mg at midnight the plasma cortisol will normally fall to very low levels when measured at 8 am the next morning.

A carefully collected salivary cortisol level may be substituted for the plasma test if the latter is inconvenient. A normal response is sufficient to rule out Cushing syndrome in the great majority of patients with suspicious clinical features. Confirmation may be obtained by a normal 24-hour urinary-free cortisol.

● Some patients without Cushing's syndrome may fail the screening test if they are obese, depressed, alcoholic, or taking medications that accelerate the metabolism of dexamethasone such as phenytoin, rifampin, carbamazine, and barbiturates.

Under these circumstances, the full 2-day low-dose test may be used to distinguish the Cushing's syndrome patients from those without the syndrome. Those patients on drugs that speed the metabolism of dexamethasone will require other testing strategy or the measurement of dexamethasone levels followed by dose adjustments of the offending agents or the dexamethasone.

● In patients who fail the low dose tests (establishing the presence of Cushing's syndrome) the high-dose test is employed to distinguish Cushing's disease (suppressible) from the ectopic ACTH syndrome (not suppressible).

Confirmation of a pituitary adenoma is by MRI and occasionally by petrosal vein sampling if imaging is not revealing.

● Adrenal adenomas and carcinomas are ACTH independent forms of Cushing's syndrome; ACTH levels are suppressed in these unilateral adrenal forms of the disease.

Imaging shows an adrenal mass. In the case of carcinomas the mass is usually very large at presentation. The contralateral adrenal is suppressed in these cases, so steroid replacement is required after surgical removal of the adrenal tumor until the other side recovers. An obligate period of subphysiologic cortisol levels is needed to permit recovery, and frequently this period is very long.

🔵 Most carcinomas do not produce Cushing's syndrome; the tumor is
an oncologic problem. When carcinomas produce excess cortisol
adrenal androgens are always increased as well, usually markedly so.

Adrenal androgens are best assessed by measuring 17-ketosteroids in a 24-hour
urine sample. In sharp contrast adrenal adenomas do not produce excess adrenal
androgens.

🔵 Physical stigmata of Cushing's syndrome that are particularly useful
include broad purple striae and proximal muscle weakness.

Obese hirsute woman with polycystic ovarian syndrome, for example, have
narrow pink striae and very good muscle strength.

🔵 The well-known physical stigmata of Cushing's syndrome are frequently
absent in the ectopic ACTH syndrome; instead of weight gain with
striae and central obesity, hypokalemic alkalosis and hyperpigmentation are frequent features at presentation.

The very high levels of ACTH found in the classic ectopic ACTH syndrome
have alpha-melanocyte–stimulating hormone activity that produces hyperpigmentation. The hypokalemic alkalosis is also secondary to the very high ACTH
levels which stimulate the adrenals to produce a variety of nonaldosterone mineralocorticoids. Type 2 diabetes mellitus may be noted as well in the ectopic
ACTH syndrome due to glucocorticoid-induced insulin resistance.

The usual stigmata of Cushing's syndrome are absent in the ectopic ACTH
syndrome because of weight loss rather than weight gain and because the manifestations develop much more quickly than in the other forms of Cushing's
syndrome.

In the ectopic ACTH syndrome secondary to small bronchial carcinoid
tumors, which grow slowly and have ACTH levels similar to those seen in
classic pituitary Cushing's syndrome the clinical manifestations resemble those
of classic Cushing's disease rather than those of the ectopic ACTH syndrome.

🔵 The ectopic ACTH syndrome is usually associated with neuroendo-
crine tumors, classically with small cell carcinoma of the lung.

Although many different tumors appear to make ACTH, the very high levels associated with the ectopic ACTH syndrome are the product of tumors derived from
neuroendocrine cells. Thus, small cell carcinoma of the lung (most common),
bronchial, and thymic carcinoids, medullary carcinoma of the thyroid, islet cell
tumors of the pancreas, and pheochromocytomas have all been associated with
the ectopic ACTH syndrome.

Bartter's Syndrome

In 1962, Frederick Bartter's described a syndrome of hypokalemia, alkalosis,
hyperreninemia, and juxtaglomerular hyperplasia in patients with normal
blood pressure. The initial hypotheses generated to explain the pathophysiology

considered reduced responsiveness to the pressor effects of angiotensin II versus deficient renal sodium conservation. Subsequent studies and eventually genetic analyses confirmed renal tubular defects as the cause.

> **Bartter's syndrome and the related Gitelman's syndrome are autosomal recessive traits that impair renal sodium reabsorption resulting in volume depletion and secondary aldosteronism with consequent hypokalemic alkalosis.**

Bartter's syndrome results from defective sodium reabsorption in the thick ascending limb of the loop of Henle, an abnormality that reflects a genetic alteration in the chloride channel. Gitelman's syndrome, which is actually a lot more common, is due to a defect in the sodium chloride cotransporter of the distal tubule. Thus, Bartter's syndrome acts as a loop diuretic and Gitelman's syndrome as a thiazide. Both diseases are associated with impaired concentrating ability. Gitelman's syndrome is associated with magnesium wasting and hypomagnesemia as well.

> **Is it Bartter's syndrome or diuretic abuse? Answer: almost always diuretic abuse.**

Bartter's syndrome is very rare and most patients presenting with hypokalemic alkalosis in whom Bartter's syndrome is suspected will turn out to have surreptitious diuretic usage.

> **The differential diagnosis of hypokalemic alkalosis includes (in addition to Bartter's and Gitelman's syndromes); primary hyperaldosteronism; secondary aldosteronism; ectopic ACTH syndrome; surreptitious diuretic use; and protracted vomiting (gastric alkalosis).**

Understanding the pathophysiology makes distinctions among these obvious in most cases. In primary aldosteronism the blood pressure is elevated and plasma renin is suppressed. In secondary aldosteronism the renin is elevated and the blood pressure is normal or high depending on the underlying cause (low or normal in cirrhosis, high in malignant hypertension). In the ectopic ACTH syndrome renin is suppressed, aldosterone is suppressed and mineralocorticoids other than aldosterone are elevated in conjunction with high ACTH levels, hypertension and a high incidence of diabetes mellitus. Gastric alkalosis from vomiting or nasogastric suction is associated with a low urinary chloride.

> **Diuretic abuse should be suspected in young women with eating disorders and in health care workers.**

Confirmation is from analysis of the urine for diuretics. Clues to the diagnosis include very low body mass index (BMI), excessive exercise, and the use of eye make-up and lipstick in the hospital.

Anorexia Nervosa

Anorexia nervosa, with or without associated bulimia, is a potentially serious psychiatric disease with issues related to control and body image. Severe cases have hypotension and bradycardia due to diminished sympathetic tone.

 Most common in young women, clues to the diagnosis of anorexia nervosa on physical examination include relatively preserved breasts despite severe inanition and fine lanugo hair over the body. If bulimia is present parotid hypertrophy from inflammation of Stensen duct and erosion of tooth enamel may be noted.

Surreptitious diuretic usage may be present as well and should be suspected in the presence of electrolyte disturbance.

Fever, Temperature Regulation, and Thermogenesis

8

CHAPTER

CENTRAL REGULATION OF CORE
TEMPERATURE

FEVER AND HYPERTHERMIA

THERMOGENESIS

HEAT GENERATION AND
DISSIPATION

DIURNAL VARIATION IN
TEMPERATURE

NIGHT SWEATS

CENTRAL REGULATION OF CORE TEMPERATURE

Temperature in humans is controlled by the hypothalamus around a set point of about 37 °C (98.6 °F), by a complex series of mechanisms that permit the generation, conservation, and dissipation of heat.

Homeothermy requires a balance of heat generation, heat conservation, and heat dissipation. This is accomplished by a remarkable series of coordinated cardiovascular and metabolic responses integrated in the hypothalamus, and fine tuned in the effector organs peripherally. These responses involve the autonomic nervous system, the skeletal musculature, arteries and veins, the sweat glands, and brown adipose tissue (BAT).

FEVER AND HYPERTHERMIA

Fever represents a resetting of the temperature set point up; antipyretics adjust the set point down when the latter is elevated by fever.

Fever is distinct from hyperthermia.

In hyperthermia the core temperature rises because heat dissipation mechanisms are impaired, or because heat production exceeds the capacity of heat dissipation mechanisms, not because of an increase in central temperature set point.

Infections cause fever via cytokine release from inflammatory cells.

In fact, the first cytokine described was called "endogenous pyrogen" since it was released from host leukocytes after exposure to bacteria. It had previously been thought that bacterial products *per se* caused the fever. Cytokines released from tumor cells also cause the fever that is associated with malignancy.

THERMOGENESIS

🔘 **Thermogenesis, literally heat production, is not synonymous with fever.**

In warm-blooded mammals (homeotherms) basal heat production (or basal metabolic rate [BMR]) is the heat produced at rest by mitochondria throughout the body. BMR is regulated by thyroid hormones.

🔘 **Excessive sweating is the clinical manifestation of increased heat production without a rise in temperature.**

In hyperthyroidism BMR is increased (thermogenesis), but fever is absent unless the increased heat production overwhelms the heat dissipation mechanisms.

HEAT GENERATION AND DISSIPATION

🔘 **Heat dissipation mechanisms include sweating and vasodilation.**

Vasodilation results in the loss of heat through the skin by radiation; sweating cools via evaporative heat loss. The latter is regulated by cholinergic sympathetic nerves to the sweat glands.

🔘 **A rise in temperature of 1 °C results in a 10% to 13% increase in metabolic rate, contributing to the weight loss noted during prolonged febrile illness.**

Maintenance of normal body temperature in spite of differing ambient conditions (homeothermy, the "warm blooded" state) consumes a significant amount of total energy production (about 50% in normally active man).

🔘 **Rigors reflect the rapidity of a rise in temperature; they are not specific for any particular cause of the fever.**

Heat generation occurs by the muscular activity induced by shivering; as the temperature rises during febrile illness episodes of shivering are experienced as rigors. **It is a *faux pearl* that rigors are caused principally by gram-negative bacterial infections.**

🔘 **BAT is a heat-generating organ.**

Although the role for BAT in physiologic heat production in small mammals and human neonates has been well accepted, BAT was long dismissed as irrelevant in adult humans. BAT has now been resuscitated and is generally recognized as functional in many adults. **It is a *faux pearl* that BAT is neither present nor functional in older humans.** A potential role for BAT (or lack thereof) in the pathogenesis of obesity is under investigation.

The production of metabolic heat in BAT is regulated by the sympathetic nervous system which turns on BAT metabolism by a β-3 receptor-mediated process. In the presence of uncoupling protein (UCP), BAT mitochondria become uncoupled so that substrate oxidation results in the production of heat rather than the synthesis of ATP. The location of BAT around the great vessels in the thorax facilitates distribution of the generated heat throughout the body. Heat production in BAT is markedly enhanced by chronic cold exposure, a process known as cold acclimation; in the cold acclimated state metabolic heat replaces the need to shiver during cold exposure.

In humans the extremities play an important role in temperature regulation.

Heat conservation occurs via vasoconstriction of arteries and superficial veins in the extremities. Venoconstriction, particularly in the superficial veins of the extremities, is mediated by α-2 adrenergic receptors, while the deep veins, which form a plexus around the arteries in the extremities, are more heavily endowed with α-1 receptors. External cooling decreases α-1 receptor affinity for NE in deep veins but increases α-2 affinity in the superficial veins, favoring a shift of blood to the deep venous system. The deep veins form a plexus around the arteries that supply the extremities, thus providing the anatomic basis for a countercurrent heat exchange mechanism. These vascular changes efficiently return heat from the arterial system perfusing the extremities to the central vascular compartment. The opposite vascular changes potentiate heat dissipation in a warm environment or when exercise necessitates heat loss.

When prescribing antipyretics it is preferable to dose the drugs at a regular interval rather than PRN for a rise in temperature, in order to avoid repeated heat generation and diaphoresis as the antipyretic wears off and is readministered.

During a febrile response heat is both conserved and generated, thereby raising the core temperature. Paradoxically, the patient feels cold since the core temperature is below the new (febrile) set point. When the fever breaks, either through resolution of the infection or the administration of antipyretics, heat is dissipated by vasodilation and sweating; the patient, paradoxically, feels warm, the core temperature now being above the normal set point.

DIURNAL VARIATION IN TEMPERATURE

Typically, fever peaks in the evening and diminishes in the morning, constituting a single daily spike.

Some diseases, however, are characterized by unusual fever patterns.

In Adult Still's disease (juvenile rheumatoid arthritis [JRA]) two daily spikes are common.

JRA is an important cause of undiagnosed febrile illness in adults. It is a difficult diagnosis to establish since the manifestations are nonspecific (arthralgias, fever, sore throat) and the characteristic rash is frustratingly evanescent. Inflammatory markers are typically very high (WBC, platelet count, ferritin level).

> **In malaria the classical pattern of every other day or every third day fever spike is not established early in the disease, so daily spikes are the rule at the time of presentation.**

Patients returning from an indigenous area with high spiking fever, headache, and malaise should be suspected of having malaria, especially if they have not taken appropriate prophylaxis.

> **In patients with a prolonged febrile illness that defies diagnosis the cause is usually malignancy.**

Hospitalized patients with undiagnosed fever despite repeated cultures and imaging will usually be found to have an occult malignancy rather than an occult infection.

NIGHT SWEATS

Why do febrile (and nonfebrile) patients sweat at night?

> **During sleep the core temperature falls almost 0.5 °C; to meet the lowered central set point, heat dissipation mechanisms are activated resulting in sweating and vasodilation.**

Although the temperature is falling paradoxically the patient feels hot (since the actual temperature is above the lowered set point).

Infectious Diseases

The clinical problem posited most often in a febrile patient: Is an infection present? If so, where is the likely site and what is the likely organism? If not infectious, what is the cause?

FEVER OF UNKNOWN ORIGIN

Prolonged fevers (greater than 101 °F for 2 to 3 weeks) that defy diagnosis utilizing state of the art testing are much less common now than in past decades, largely because of better imaging modalities and improved microbiologic techniques that better identify occult infections. Interestingly, however, the fundamental causes have remained amazingly similar: infections (including tuberculosis [TB]); malignancies (predominantly, lymphoproliferative diseases); and collagen vascular (autoimmune diseases).

 When an exhaustive search for infection is negative occult malignancy is the usual cause of prolonged unidentified fevers.

It should be pointed out, however, that some patients recover completely with no cause identified and others recur and still defy diagnosis. Extrapulmonary TB needs to be considered in patients with prolonged fevers that defy identification.

INFECTIONS OF SPECIFIC SITES

Urinary Tract and Kidney

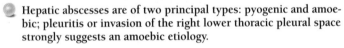 **Lower urinary tract infections (cystitis) are associated with frequency and dysuria, but not fever; fever indicates pyelonephritis.**

Acute pyelonephritis may take 72 hours to respond to antibiotics, but in general is not a serious disease particularly in young women. The usual organisms are gastrointestinal (GI) bacteria commonly *Escherichia coli, or Klebsiella.*

Repeated attacks of pyelonephritis require evaluation for structural urinary tract abnormalities.

In men pyelonephritis suggests obstruction, usually, prostatic hypertrophy.

A positive urine culture for *Staphylococcus aureus* signifies staphylococcal bacteremia and has the same significance as a positive blood culture.

Although staph may secondarily infect the kidneys, a positive urine culture for should not be ascribed to primary kidney infection.

Sterile pyuria raises the question of genitourinary TB.

The renal collecting system is not an uncommon site of extrapulmonary TB. Hematuria is also common in genitourinary TB, and calcifications may be noted in the collecting system on x-ray.

Liver

Hepatic abscesses are of two principal types: pyogenic and amoebic; pleuritis or invasion of the right lower thoracic pleural space strongly suggests an amoebic etiology.

Traditionally difficult to diagnose and an important cause of undiagnosed febrile illness, advanced imaging techniques have made recognition of liver abscess relatively easy, although early in the course of disease these techniques may not be diagnostic. Elevation of the right hemidiaphragm on chest x-ray may suggest the diagnosis.

Pyogenic abscesses are usually a consequence of a septic focus in the abdomen or the biliary system. Anaerobic organisms are frequently involved.

Amoebic abscess is a consequence of colonic infection, principally in the cecum, and may follow a bout of amoebic hepatitis.

Portal drainage of the cecum preferentially delivers blood to the posterior aspect of the right lobe explaining the predominant location of amoebic abscesses in the right lobe posteriorly. Secondary infection of amoebic abscesses with pyogenic anaerobic bacteria is not unusual. Prompt catheter drainage is required in addition to appropriate antibiotic treatment.

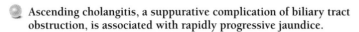 Ascending cholangitis, a suppurative complication of biliary tract obstruction, is associated with rapidly progressive jaundice.

Biliary stones in the common bile duct are the most common cause, but strictures and carcinomas (ampullary, pancreatic, and cholangiocarcinoma) may be complicated by cholangitis as well. Cholangitis is said to be "ascending" because the biliary tract, usually sterile, is infected by invading organisms from the gut in the presence of obstruction. The responsible organisms are usually gut flora, aerobic gram-negative rods, especially *E. coli* and *Klebsiella*. The constellation of right upper quadrant pain, fever, and jaundice (Charcot's triad) suggests the diagnosis, but the key is rapidly progressive jaundice. Anaerobic organisms, usual in hepatic abscesses, are not common in biliary infections.

Acute viral hepatitis is associated with malaise, anorexia, nausea, low-grade fever, icteric skin and eyes, dark urine, and right upper quadrant tenderness. The WBC is never elevated (usually 7,000) and the differential reveals 50% polys and 50% mononuclear cells.

In smokers a loss of taste for cigarettes may be an early symptom.

Hepatitis A virus (HAV) occurs in point source epidemics involving fecal contamination of water or shellfish and may (rarely) cause severe injury with hepatic failure requiring a liver transplant; it is a not a cause of chronic liver disease. Hepatitis B virus (HBV) and hepatitis C virus (HCV) are blood-borne infections usually acquired from contaminated blood products or needles or through sexual contact. HBV and HCV may result in chronic infection and cirrhosis as well as hepatocellular carcinoma. Collapse of the normal hepatic portal architecture with necrosis that bridges the portal triads predicts the subsequent development of cirrhosis.

The immunologic response to HBV and especially HCV may result in mixed essential cryoglobulinemia.

Vaccination has significantly reduced the incidence of HAV and HBV.

Epstein–Barr virus (EBV) and cytomegalovirus (CMV) may also cause hepatitis.

These infections characteristically cause a mild hepatitis, although CMV infections may be prolonged even in immunocompetent patients.

Spine and Epidural Space

Back pain and fever strongly suggest the diagnosis of spinal epidural abscess.

An epidural collection of pus that threatens spinal cord compression, spinal epidural abscess should be ruled out in every case of back pain that presents with fever. MRI is the preferred imaging modality.

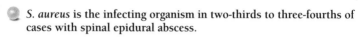

- **S. aureus is the infecting organism in two-thirds to three-fourths of cases with spinal epidural abscess.**

Hematogenous dissemination is the usual method of infection, although spread from contiguous infection in a vertebrae or disc also occurs. Skin or soft tissue infection is thought to be the usual portal of entry, although in a significant portion of cases no site can be identified.

- **Other organisms responsible for epidural abscess include streptococci, particularly group B strep, gram-negative rods, nocardia, fungi, and mycobacterium TB.**

Lumbar puncture is contraindicated because of the possibility of spread of the infecting organism. The thoracolumbar spine is the most common area involved. Elderly men are most commonly affected and diabetes increases the susceptibility. Tenderness to palpation is usually, but not always, present.

- **Signs of cord compression (leg weakness, incontinence, and a sensory level) indicate the need for immediate decompression of the epidural abscess by laminectomy and debridement.**

The administration of antibiotics should begin as soon as the diagnosis is established by MRI and operative intervention is needed at the first sign of cord compression.

- **Vertebral osteomyelitis and discitis present with fever and back pain.**

The pathogenesis of vertebral and disc infection is similar to spinal epidural abscess, and **S. aureus** is the common infecting bacteria. Unlike epidural abscess antibiotics are sufficient for treatment and surgical debridement is not required unless the imaging or clinical findings suggest cord compression.

- **Tuberculous involvement of the spine frequently involves adjacent vertebrae and the intervening disc space.**

- **A psoas abscess may complicate tuberculous or pyogenic infection of the spine or epidural space. A positive "psoas sign" may be useful diagnostically.**

Extension of the hip with the leg straight, in the lateral position with the involved side up, tests for a psoas sign; the latter is positive when pain is elicited as the leg is extended at the hip. It is also useful in detecting retrocecal appendicitis as the inflamed appendix abuts the psoas muscle.

Pharyngitis

- **Group A streptococci and EBV (infectious mononucleosis) both cause acute pharyngitis, tender cervical lymphadenopathy, and fever; they may be difficult to distinguish on the basis of physical examination, but can easily be differentiated by associated clinical and laboratory features. Both infections may occasionally coexist.**

Both strep and mono may have extensive exudate, tonsillar enlargement, and very erythematous pharyngeal mucosa. Mono frequently has palatal petechiae and an edematous uvula.

🔵 **Vomiting is common with strep throat. Splenomegaly is common with mono.**

🔵 **CBC with differential easily distinguishes the two: strep throat has a leukocytosis with granulocyte predominance; mono has normal or elevated WBC with many mononuclear cells including (frequently) atypical lymphocytes (Downey cells) which are cytotoxic T cells directed against infected B lymphocytes.**

The "monospot" test, successor to the Paul–Bunnell heterophile agglutinin test, is quite specific for mono, but lacks sensitivity especially early in the course of the disease and is negative in the month-long incubation period. It must be kept in mind that strep and mono may coexist, so a low threshold for a strep screen in patients with mono is a reasonable idea.

🔵 **If ampicillin (or amoxicillin) is given to a patient with mono it is almost certain that a rash will develop; such a rash, however, does not necessarily indicate drug allergy.**

🔵 **The hepatitis associated with EBV in immunocompetent patients is characteristically mild and not associated with chronic liver disease.**

Lung Abscess

🔵 **There are several different types of lung abscess; the common feature is necrosis of pulmonary parenchyma caused by microbial infection.**

The major causes of pulmonary infection with necrosis are: 1) aspiration of oropharyngeal (particularly dental) flora; 2) suppuration and necrosis in an area of acute bacterial pneumonia; 3) secondary infection in a necrotic area of lung as a complication of bronchogenic carcinoma, collagen vascular disease (particularly Wegener's granulomatosis), or pulmonary embolus with infarction; and 4) metastatic infection from hematogenous dissemination of an infectious process in another region of the body.

🔵 **The classic lung abscess is in an indolent anaerobic infection from aspiration of mouth flora. Alcoholic stupor is an important predisposing factor.**

Symptoms develop over weeks to months; the patient is chronically ill with fever, cough, and the production of purulent fetid sputum. The feculent smell is indicative of anaerobic infection, especially anaerobic streptococci.

🔵 **Clubbing may be present in patients with lung abscess.**

Chest x-ray shows a cavity with an air fluid level. Treatment is a prolonged course (months) of antibiotics with effective anaerobic coverage. Surgical drainage is not required for two reasons: 1) communication with the airway permits discharge of the contents; and 2) the compliance of lung tissue avoids the buildup of pressure within the cavity and permits adequate antibiotic penetration.

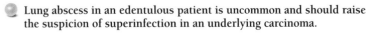 **Lung abscess in an edentulous patient is uncommon and should raise the suspicion of superinfection in an underlying carcinoma.**

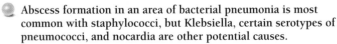 **Abscess formation in an area of bacterial pneumonia is most common with staphylococci, but Klebsiella, certain serotypes of pneumococci, and nocardia are other potential causes.**

Bowel Infections

The causes of infectious gastroenteritis are legion and include pathogens of bacterial, viral, and protozoan origin.

Fecal–oral transmission and contaminated food and water account for the spread of most bowel infections.

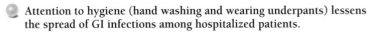 **Attention to hygiene (hand washing and wearing underpants) lessens the spread of GI infections among hospitalized patients.**

Viral Gastroenteritis

Viral gastroenteritis causes vomiting and nonbloody diarrhea, is usually mild, and is almost always short lived; it is the most common infectious disease of the gut. Norovirus is the most common etiologic agent among the viruses that cause gastroenteritis.

The illness lasts 1 to 2 days although some severe norovirus infections may last longer. Norovirus derives its name from an outbreak in Norwalk, Ohio; it was found to be filterable, and therefore nonbacterial, and referred to as the "Norwalk agent" before the virus was identified.

BACTERIAL GASTROENTERITIS

Campylobacter, certain subtypes of *E. Coli, Salmonella,* and *Shigella,* all gram-negative rods, are the most common bacterial pathogens causing gastroenteritis. Diagnosis is established by culturing the organism from the stool. *Clostridium difficile* and *S. aureus,* gram-positive organisms, produce toxins that inflame the bowel and cause diarrhea.

Salmonella

Salmonella infection in humans produces a spectrum of GI disease that varies from acute gastroenteritis at one end to enteric fever at the other.

Salmonella enteritis at one extreme may cause an afebrile, nonbloody, self-limited diarrheal disease; at the other a serious invasive infection of the small and large bowel with fever, toxicity, and with local (and distal) complications. In reality, the distinction between the benign enteritis and enteric fever is usually blurred; the disease caused by salmonella in humans represents a continuous spectrum from mild gastroenteritis to severe enteric fever.

- **Unlike other Salmonella species, which are endemic in warm- and cold-blooded animals, S. Typhi is an obligate human pathogen. Typhoid fever is contracted from infected patients or chronic carriers.**

Typhoid fever is the prototypical enteric fever. Although uncommon in the United States at present, typhoid is common worldwide and should be suspected in patients with febrile illnesses returning from areas where the infection is endemic (parts of Southeast Asia, the Middle East, Africa, and Latin America).

- **Unlike typhoid fever which is rare in the United States, Salmonella enteritis is a common form of food-borne illness ("food poisoning").**

The severity of the disease varies greatly but many cases are characterized by fever, abdominal pain, and diarrhea which may be bloody. Improperly handled poultry is a common source of infection with non-*S. typhi* strains. Outbreaks of varying size may occur from a contaminated source at a social event. Stool cultures are positive and blood cultures may be positive as well. The systemic manifestations reflect the impact of endotoxin release and are most marked in the enteric fever form of the infection.

- **The presence of fever, blood, and leukocytes in the stool indicates invasive disease requiring treatment with antibiotics.**

Invasive salmonella infections are frequently associated with bacteremia and should be treated with the appropriate antibiotic, ceftriaxone. **The contention that antibiotics should be avoided in cases of (non-*S. typhi*) salmonella enteritis because treatment may result in a prolonged carrier state is a *faux pearl*, often cited by infectious disease specialists.** It makes no sense since nontyphoid strains of salmonella are not associated with prolonged carriage, and typhoid fever, which may be, is always treated with antibiotics.

- **Typhoid fever is not associated with diarrhea in the early phases of the disease.**

Fever and abdominal pain dominate the clinical picture of early typhoid fever; splenomegaly and a characteristic rash (rose spots) may be present along with leukopenia and bradycardia (despite fever). Intestinal perforation is a feared complication since the organisms heavily infect the Peyer's patches in the ileum. The patient should be kept NPO until the symptoms resolve and then the reintroduction of feeding should be slow and cautious. (Alexander the Great is said to have died of intestinal perforation in Babylon on his return from India, apparently because he was fed too early – chicken – in the recovery phase of an illness that was very likely typhoid fever).

Salmonella bacteremia (non–*S. typhi* strains) has a predilection for secondarily infecting atheromatous arteries.

Metastatic infection may involve existing abdominal aneurysms or cause mycotic aneurysms.

Relapsing salmonella bacteremia or persistently positive blood cultures should raise suspicion of an endovascular site of infection.

Campylobacter

The most common cause of bacterial gastroenteritis in adults, infection with *Campylobacter jejuni* causes an acute diarrheal syndrome that may be bloody, and that may be followed by reactive arthritis (Reiter's syndrome) or an immune-mediated polyradiculoneuropathy (Guillain–Barre syndrome).

The clinical features of campylobacter infection and the factors that predispose to infection are similar to those of salmonella gastroenteritis. There is an animal reservoir of campylobacter and undercooked poultry is a common source of infection.

The association with Guillain–Barre is likely an example of "molecular mimicry" with antibodies to campylobacter antigens cross-reacting to epitopes on myelin.

Shigella

Shigellosis, also known as bacillary dysentery, is an infection of the distal colon and rectum. The major features reflect the distal localization of the lesions: urgency, tenesmus, scant bloody diarrhea, and cramping abdominal pain.

The pathogenesis involves direct mucosal invasion and production of Shiga toxin which damages the mucosal colonic epithelium. Rectal swab should be performed as well as stool culture as this enhances the likelihood of culturing the organism.

Pathogenic *Escherichia coli*

Long known as normal gut flora, over the last several decades it has become increasingly recognized that some *E. coli* subtypes possess substantial pathogenetic potential; these are now recognized as an important cause of bacterial enterocolitis.

The clinical manifestations of *E. coli* enterocolitis depend upon the virulence factors acquired by the particular subtype. The only subtype that can be identified in routine clinical practice is O157, the strain that produces Shiga toxin.

Shiga producing strains of *E. coli*, particularly, O157:H7 have been strongly implicated in the pathogenesis of the hemolytic uremic syndrome (HUS).

These strains are known as enterohemorrhagic *E. coli* as they produce severe bloody diarrhea.

Enterotoxigenic *E. coli* are not invasive but cause a watery nonbloody diarrhea; they are a prominent cause of "traveler's diarrhea." The toxins elaborated stimulate intestinal secretion by an adenylate cyclase/cyclic AMP mechanism and are distinct from the Shiga toxins that are associated with severe invasive disease. Enteroinvasive strains of *E. coli* cause a more severe colitis akin to those caused by Shigella.

Clostridium difficile (C. diff)

Certain strains of these anaerobic, spore-forming, gram-positive rods elaborate toxins that cause diarrhea and, occasionally, severe colitis with pseudomembrane formation. *C. diff* is not invasive and strains that do not produce the toxins do not cause disease. Antibiotics potentiate colonization of the colon with *C. diff* which is the major cause of antibiotic-associated diarrhea.

 C. diff **classically causes colitis in hospitalized patients on antibiotics. Despite the fact that the infection is not invasive fever, abdominal pain and leukocytosis are frequently noted.**

The diagnosis is established not by culture but by demonstration of the *C. diff* toxin in the stool.

 Clindamycin was the first antibiotic implicated in *C. diff* **colitis and remains an important cause but it is now recognized that a wide variety of antibiotics including the fluoroquinolones and the beta-lactams are commonly implicated.**

Cancer chemotherapy predisposes as well.

 Along with antibiotic usage hospitalization was previously considered a prerequisite for *C. diff* **diarrhea; it is now recognized that many patients acquire the disease in the community, some without a history of antibiotic usage.**

Occasional cases are quite severe and unresponsive to treatment. In these patients colectomy was a last resort but recently fecal transplants to restore normal bowel flora have shown promise.

Staphylococcal Enterotoxin Enteritis

S. aureus produces an exotoxin (enterotoxin B) which is an important cause of "food poisoning."

 Staphylococcal food poisoning begins 1 to 8 hours after eating contaminated food and is characterized by vomiting and diarrhea, both often explosive. The symptoms are short lived, usually ending in less than 12 hours.

The pathogenesis involves the ingestion of preformed toxin generated by staphylococci multiplying in improperly refrigerated food, classically mayonnaise in chicken or tuna salad in hot weather, and at picnics.

Staphylococcal enterotoxin B is also the cause of some nonmenstrual staphylococcal toxic shock syndromes.

SPECIFIC INFECTIOUS AGENTS

Gonococci (GC)

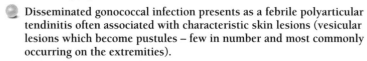 **Disseminated gonococcal infection presents as a febrile polyarticular tendinitis often associated with characteristic skin lesions (vesicular lesions which become pustules – few in number and most commonly occurring on the extremities).**

This is the bacteremic phase of the disease.

The bacteremic phase of disseminated gonococcal infection may be followed by the development of typical septic arthritis in one or two large joints.

Arthrocentesis at this latter stage reveals large numbers of polys and it may be possible to culture the organism from the joint fluid.

Disseminated GC is much more common in women and typically occurs in the perimenstrual period or in early pregnancy when the normal endometrial barrier to dissemination is compromised.

The asymptomatic carrier state, the reservoir for dissemination, is not uncommon in women but does not occur in men.

In the early phase of the disseminated form of GC the response to intravenous antibiotics is prompt with rapid resolution of fever and tendinitis.

The rapid response to therapy helps secure the diagnosis.

Meningococci

Acute infections with the meningococcus, meningococcemia, and meningococcal meningitis, are well known serious diseases, endemic in sub-Saharan Africa and frequently occurring in epidemics in the United States, particularly in overcrowded areas and among military recruits.

Chronic meningococcemia is a rare disease characterized by recurrent bouts of fever, headache, chills, arthralgias, anorexia, occasionally diarrhea or vomiting, and an erythematous maculopapular or petechial eruption on the extremities and occasionally on the trunk.

Chronic meningococcemia is a curious disease since meningococcemia is almost always acute and fulminant with shock, disseminated intravascular coagulation, a petechial eruption that evolves into purplish ecchymosis, and, not uncommonly, adrenal hemorrhage which contributes to the shock (Waterhouse–Friedrichsen syndrome). The typical acute presentation is a consequence of endotoxin release which results in a thrombohemorrhagic state (DIC) reminiscent of a general Schwartzman reaction. Meningococcal meningitis is frequently associated. It is not known why some patients have a chronic form of the disease nor why chronic nasopharyngeal carriage of meningococci does not more frequently result in acute disease. Chronic meningococcemia, however, may devolve into the acute septicemic form or meningitis, so recognition and treatment are critical.

> **The typical case of chronic meningococcemia presents to the emergency room with fever, rash, headache, malaise, and anorexia. There is frequently a history of similar episodes in the recent past.**

Absent localizing signs the patient is sent home for outpatient follow–up, but because the patient does not appear well and is febrile blood cultures are drawn. When these are returned positive for pleomorphic gram negative diplococci, to the alarm of the ER staff, the patient is called back, admitted and appropriate treatment initiated.

Staphylococcal Infections

> **Staphylococcal bacteremia is the proximate cause of infection of the joints and the heart valves as well as the vertebrae and epidural space.**

The portal of entry for the bacteremia is thought to be the skin or soft tissue but often no nidus of infection is detected. The bacteremia itself may be associated with diarrhea perhaps related to a staphylococcal toxin. Urine culture may be positive for Staph as the bacteria are filtered in the kidney. Prompt treatment is necessary to prevent multiple long term complications.

> **Staphylococci are an important cause of acute bacterial endocarditis which is frequently associated with rapid valve destruction, embolization, and congestive failure.**

Prompt surgical intervention is usually required. Interestingly, prognosis appears to be better in intravenous drug abusers where the portal of entry is contaminated needles, rather than in patients without a drug history.

> **Toxic shock syndrome, a serious complication of staphylococcal infection, is due to the elaboration of a toxin which causes fever, diffuse erythema, hypotension, and in severe cases, multi-organ system failure.**

First recognized in menstruating women using super absorbent tampons it is now recognized that staphylococcal infection at different sites may be responsible for elaborating the toxin that is responsible for the syndrome. Cases may follow influenza with staphylococcal superinfection, childbirth, or sinus infection, as well as vaginal infection associated with tampon use. Intensive treatment of the hypotension and eradicating the source of the infection are the therapeutic goals.

> Streptococcal toxic shock, secondary to a related toxin elaborated in group A β-hemolytic strep infections, is more serious than classic staphylococcal toxic shock syndrome, is more commonly associated with renal failure, and a higher mortality rate.

The common portal of entry is skin infection or necrotizing fasciitis.

Syphilis (Lues)

Sexually transmitted, this spirochetal disease begins with the characteristic painless firm ulceration on the penis or cervix. If untreated secondary lues appears 2 weeks to 3 months after the primary infection.

> It is important to recognize secondary syphilis since in many cases a history of primary infection is absent and the secondary phase is highly infectious.

The typical patient presents with a rash, malaise, lymphadenopathy, sometimes with fever and arthralgias. Skin lesions (and occasionally mucosal lesions) are the key to the diagnosis but these may be variable in appearance. Violaceous to brown depending on the region of the body and the complexion of the patient, these maculopapular, squamous, occasionally scaling lesions may appear on the trunk or the extremities or on the palms and soles.

> Location of luetic lesions on the palms and soles is highly suspicious and usually the key to the diagnosis.

A high index of suspicion is required.

> The secondary luetic lesions are swarming with spirochetes and hence very infectious, especially the moist lesions on mucosal surfaces.

> Every patient with a sexually transmitted disease should have a sero-logic test for syphilis.

> Treatment of secondary syphilis with penicillin may result in the Jarisch–Herxheimer reaction, a consequence of the rapid killing of large numbers of organisms with the release of proinflammatory cytokines.

Fever, chills, hypotension, and apprehension may be severe necessitating intravenous fluids and in some cases glucocorticoids.

> Luetic aortitis, a form of tertiary syphilis, occurring years after the initial infection, involves the ascending aorta; aneurysmal dilatation is the consequence which may be associated with aortic regurgitation.

Aortic regurgitation in luetic aneurysm is best heard over the right precordium at the second intercostal space and is associated with a "booming" (tambour) aortic closure sound.

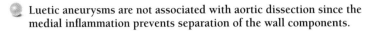 Luetic aneurysms are not associated with aortic dissection since the medial inflammation prevents separation of the wall components.

The aneurysms may, however, be quite large.

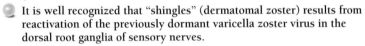 Tabes dorsalis is a luetic myelopathy, a tertiary form of neurosyphilis involving the posterior columns of the spinal cord.

It is associated with parasthesias (shooting "lightning" pains) and extensive loss of proprioception. It may be associated with destructive arthritis of the knee (Charcot joint).

Herpes Zoster

It is well recognized that "shingles" (dermatomal zoster) results from reactivation of the previously dormant varicella zoster virus in the dorsal root ganglia of sensory nerves.

After the childhood exanthem chickenpox the varicella zoster virus lies dormant in the dorsal root ganglia of sensory nerves. Waning immunity, as occurs with aging, the use of immunosuppressive drugs, or diseases which compromise the immune system, is associated with reactivation of the latent infection. A curious observation, largely unexplained, is that an attack of zoster in adults sometimes follows exposure to a child with chickenpox. How can this be since zoster is the reactivation of a dormant infection? Perhaps re-exposure via the respiratory tree attracts varicella antibodies to the portal of entry, thus freeing up virus previously pinned down in the dorsal root ganglia, thereby permitting emergence along the sensory nerves.

Zoster begins with pain in a dermatomal distribution followed in 2 to 3 days by erythematous macules that vesiculate, become pustular, and impetiginize.

Early treatment with antiviral agents may abort the usual progression.

Fever and a cerebrospinal fluid pleocytosis (with or without aseptic meningitis) may occur with zoster.

An episode of zoster does not require work up for an underlying malignancy beyond history, physical examination, and age-appropriate screening.

Involvement of the geniculate ganglion of the facial (VII cranial) nerve results in the Ramsay Hunt syndrome (herpes zoster oticus): pain in the ear followed by typical lesions in the external auditory canal, and, frequently, facial paresis.

The facial paralysis has a worse prognosis for recovery than the usual case of Bell's palsy. Loss of taste over the anterior two-thirds of the tongue may be associated.

Zoster ophthalmicus occurs with involvement of the first (ophthalmic) division of the V cranial nerve.

Pain often begins at the tip of the nose. Pain and inflammation of the anterior structures of the eye may threaten vision and necessitate prompt treatment.

> Tzanck smear is useful in identifying zoster or herpes simplex in vesicular lesions: multinucleate giant cells are present in scrapings from the base of vesicles.

Herpes Simplex Virus (HSV)

> In addition to the well-known fever blister (herpes labialis) herpes simplex causes mucocutaneous stomatitis, herpes genitalis, encephalitis, aseptic meningitis, keratitis, Bell's palsy, erythema multiform (Stevens–Johnson syndrome), an uncommon finger infection (herpetic whitlow), and rarely, a widely disseminated vaccinia-like rash known as Kaposi's varicelliform eruption.

> Herpes labialis, the fever blister or "cold sore," is the footprint of prior HSV type 1 infection, representing reactivation of a latent HSV-1 infection.

Typically located on the border of the upper or lower lip it may rarely involve the hard palate or gums.

> Primary HSV-1 infection occurs in children or young adults and may result in a severe but self-limited erosive ulceration of the gingiva, pharynx, and buccal mucosa.

It is accompanied by fever and malaise.

> Genital herpes is a sexually transmitted disease usually caused by HSV type 2 but may be caused by HSV-1 as well.

It is typically a painful erosive cluster of vesicles on the genitalia but may be asymptomatic. Recurrent episodes are usual, especially with HSV-2.

> Herpetic encephalitis is a serious CNS infection that may represent primary or reactivation HSV-1 disease.

Temporal lobe involvement is usual and MRI frequently shows subtle signs of bleeding in this area. The virus may be detected in the CSF. Treatment should begin promptly with IV acyclovir or its congeners.

> HSV is an important cause of viral "aseptic" meningitis. Recurrent aseptic meningitis, known as "Mollaret's syndrome" is usually caused by HSV-2.

Also known as benign recurrent lymphocytic meningitis, it is self-limited but usually treated with acyclovir.

> Corneal involvement (keratitis) by HSV-1 is severe and threatens vision. If suspected immediate ophthalmologic consultation is mandatory.

● **Herpetic whitlow is a painful erythematous, vesicular or pustular lesion of the fingertip caused by HSV-1. In immunosuppressed patients, AIDS for example, the lesion may look necrotic and resemble gangrene.**

Diagnosis is important because surgery is contraindicated and the response to acyclovir rapid and impressive.

● **Human Herpes virus 8 (HHV-8) is the cause of Kaposi's sarcoma.**

In young HIV positive adults the lesions frequently occur about the face, upper body, and internal organs; in older non-HIV patients the legs are the most common sites of involvement.

● **Kaposi's varicelliform eruption is a disseminated vesiculopustular skin infection that occurs in areas of pre-existing skin disease, most notably, atopic dermatitis. HSV is the usual cause and gives rise to the alternative name "eczema herpticum."**

This is a serious disease and may be fatal. Smallpox vaccination (vaccinia virus) may give rise to the syndrome in children with atopic dermatitis. Tzanck prep is positive but does not distinguish between HSV and zoster or vaccinia, but both are treated with acyclovir. Diagnosis is confirmed by demonstrating the herpes virus in the vesicular fluid. Other skin disease may predispose as well including pemphigus vulgaris.

● **CMV, a member of the herpes virus family is a well-recognized cause of disseminated opportunistic infection in immunosuppressed patients. In immunocompetent individuals it may cause a mono-like syndrome with fever, malaise, and fatigue.**

In distinction to EBV pharyngitis is absent. The illness in the immunocompetent may last weeks. Liver function abnormalities reflective of hepatitis are often present with fever and a predominance of mononuclear cells in the WBC differential.

GLOBALIZATION AND INFECTIOUS DISEASE

Travel history is vital in the evaluation of patients with febrile illnesses. Knowledge of infections endemic in the regions visited by returning sick travelers or immigrants is essential.

Malaria

Endemic areas include Latin America, the Middle East, Africa, and Southeast Asia. Travelers from these areas should be asked in detail about prophylactic medications and mosquito bites.

● **High spiking fever, headache, and rigors in a traveler returning from an endemic area will usually turn out to be falciparum malaria.**

At the onset the febrile spikes occur daily which may mislead. The history will usually reveal that prophylaxis was omitted or not administered properly including after return.

🔵 **TB is a serious concern in immigrants from Southeast Asia.**

Diseases that have Spread Beyond their Traditional Locales

Globalization has changed the pattern of distribution of many diseases. The recent emergence of West Nile Virus from the Middle East to become endemic in the United States and other regions is a good example. Dengue fever is another example of a tropical disease that has developed a worldwide distribution over the last half century. The recent spread of chikungunya to the western hemisphere from endemic regions in Africa and southern Asia is the latest of these diseases to spread to the United States following its initial appearance in the Caribbean. Autochthonous (indigenous) cases have been reported in Florida and more are expected as the reservoir in the animal world enlarges and the arthropod vectors spread north.

🔵 **Chikungunya fever is an arbovirus infection (spread by two species of Aedes) characterized by fever, painful arthralgias and arthritis, malaise, and a maculopapular morbilliform rash.**

The distinguishing feature is the severity of the joint manifestations which differentiates chikungunya from dengue fever. Another distinguishing point is the absence of leukopenia, common in dengue fever. The term chikungunya is from an African dialect that means "bent over" in reference to the stooped posture imposed by the joint pains. Hands and feet are most prominently involved. Although the illness is usually self-limited, lasting about 1 week, the joint pains may persist for long periods of time.

Pulmonary *10*

BLOOD GASES

Gas exchange is the principle function of the lungs which work, under the direction of the central nervous system, to maintain a partial pressure of oxygen in the blood (PaO_2) of about 90 mm Hg and a partial pressure of carbon dioxide ($PaCO_2$) of about 40 mm Hg.

Hypoxemia and Hypercapnia

 Hypoxemia has serious adverse consequences and must be treated aggressively to avoid pulmonary hypertension and right heart failure (cor pulmonale). When PaO_2 falls below 60 mm Hg, significant desaturation of hemoglobin occurs and oxygen delivery to tissues is impaired.

The pulmonary vasculature responds to low oxygen tension by vasoconstriction. This highly conserved primitive response serves the useful function of diminishing blood flow through sections of the lung that are poorly ventilated but well perfused, the so-called V/Q mismatch. By limiting flow to the poorly ventilated (hypoxic) areas vasoconstriction reduces the impact of the V/Q mismatch on systemic PaO_2.

Like every compensatory mechanism, however, there is a price to pay: in the presence of systemic hypoxemia pulmonary arterial vasoconstriction results in pulmonary hypertension and, eventually, right ventricular failure (*cor pulmonale*) since the right ventricle tolerates a pressure load poorly. The treatment is provision of supplemental oxygen to maintain the PaO_2 above 60 mm Hg.

● Tissue oxygenation is influenced by the oxygen/hemoglobin dissociation curve; when this curve is shifted to the left so that less oxygen is released at a given PaO_2, hypoxia, a deficiency of oxygen at the tissue level, may result (see Fig. 2.2).

Factors that shift the dissociation curve to the right, favoring oxygen release and therefore tissue oxygenation, include red cell 2,3-diphosphoglycerate (2,3-DPG) and systemic acidosis. These facts have implications for the treatment of diabetic ketoacidosis.

● CO_2 retention (hypercarbia or hypercapnia) is synonymous with alveolar hypoventilation.

In the absence of significant neuromuscular disease or severe obesity, chronic obstructive pulmonary disease (COPD) is the usual cause. It results in respiratory acidosis and a compensatory rise in serum bicarbonate.

● Prolonged and severe hypercapnia may be associated with a metabolic encephalopathy characterized by somnolence, asterixis, and papilledema, the latter reflective of cerebral vasodilation.

Treatment of hypoxemia in alveolar hypoventilation is essential, but supplemental oxygen must be administered judiciously (e.g., low flow oxygen at 2 L/min to achieve a PaO_2 of 60 mm Hg) as oxygen may depress respirations further and result in respiratory arrest. Obviously, sedative medications are to be avoided.

● Ondine's curse, failure of the central respiratory center, particularly during sleep, also known as primary alveolar hypoventilation, causes hypercarbia, hypoxemia, and death from respiratory failure.

Ondine was a nymph of German myth that delivered a curse to her unfaithful husband who had promised that "every waking breath" would bear testimony to his love. This is a disease of unknown cause that would result in death from respiratory failure but for a lifetime of mechanical ventilation.

Obstructive Sleep Apnea

● Obstructive sleep apnea (OSA) is an important cause of hypertension and daytime sleepiness.

Collapse of the upper airway causes stertorous breathing and gives way to apnea which may occur hundreds of times a night. The asphyxia that follows the apnea leads to repeated awakenings and disruption of normal sleep. In addition to sleepiness during the daytime, sympathetic nervous system (SNS) activity is increased substantially by OSA; this increase persists during the daytime and is an important cause of the hypertension that results from OSA since effective treatment diminishes both the sympathetic stimulation and the hypertension.

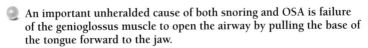

> An important unheralded cause of both snoring and OSA is failure of the genioglossus muscle to open the airway by pulling the base of the tongue forward to the jaw.

The genioglossus, which arises from the tip of the mandible and inserts on the base of the tongue, is the first respiratory muscle to contract during a respiratory cycle. Impaired function during sleep, particularly when lying supine, allows the base of the tongue to occlude the upper airway producing the sonorous noises called snoring. Most patients with OSA have a history of loud snoring but most individuals who snore do not have OSA. Alcohol, nighttime sedatives, and supine position accentuate the problem.

> Most, but not all, patients with OSA are obese. This association is probably multifactorial, but fat deposits occluding the airway and infiltrating the genioglossus are likely involved.

Interestingly, even small amounts of weight loss can produce significant improvement in OSA. Treatment is aimed at keeping the airway open by avoiding predisposing causes, and by the application of devices that deliver positive pressure to the upper airway. Mouth pieces that protrude the jaw forward and prevent the collapse of the base of the tongue have also been tried with some success. Electrical devices that stimulate the hypoglossal nerve and contract the genioglossus muscle are in clinical trials.

Hyperventilation Syndrome

> Psychogenic hyperventilation is a prominent cause of dyspnea in healthy young adults; frequent sighing is a common manifestation and should suggest the diagnosis.

Most common in anxious young healthy women, hyperventilation usually presents as dyspnea. Respiratory alkalosis is present and is frequently associated with latent tetany. Elicitation of a Chvostek sign is helpful in establishing the diagnosis. Perioral parasthesias are common as well.

> The symptoms of hyperventilation can frequently be reproduced by having the patient voluntarily overbreathe.

Hypophosphatemia and a slight rise in calcium (alkalosis increases binding to albumin) are frequently present and may initiate an unwarranted investigation for hyperparathyroidism. Hyperventilation is also a well-recognized component of panic attacks.

PULMONARY FUNCTION TESTS

> Measurement of lung volumes and expiratory flow rate distinguishes between restrictive (interstitial) and obstructive lung disease.

Investigating a patient with dyspnea begins with a chest x-ray and pulmonary function tests (PFTs). Both obstructive and restrictive lung diseases cause reduced vital capacity. Patients with interstitial lung disease have reduced lung volumes while lung volumes are increased in patients with obstructive lung disease.

🔹 **Measurement of diffusing capacity (DLCO) utilizes the affinity of hemoglobin for carbon monoxide (CO) to assess impairment of oxygen diffusion across the alveolar membrane.**

DLCO is reduced in most lung diseases including restrictive and obstructive disease. It is increased in pulmonary hemorrhage.

🔹 **An elevated DLCO, especially if marked, in a patient with changing pulmonary infiltrates is diagnostic of pulmonary hemorrhage.**

PNEUMONIA

🔹 Classifying pneumonias as "typical" or "atypical" remains useful since it provides insight into the likely infectious organism and guides appropriate treatment (Table 10-1).

Although recognition of nosocomial infection as a cause of pneumonia is obviously important, the current widely embraced classification of pneumonia as "hospital acquired" or "community acquired" is not very helpful. It is self-evident that an institutionalized, or recently institutionalized, patient needs broad spectrum coverage for those organisms likely to be acquired in hospital or nursing home. The same is true for patients who are immunocompromised either from underlying disease or medications.

TABLE 10.1 Pneumonia

"Typical" Pneumonia	"Atypical" Pneumonia
Bacterial	**Nonbacterial**
Pneumococcal (prototype)	Mycoplasma (prototype)
Hemophilus	Chlamydia
Staph	Adenovirus
Klebsiella	
Fever, shaking chill, productive cough, pleuritic pain	Fever, dyspnea, malaise, headache, dry cough
On PE: rales, dullness, + egophony, ↑ fremitus	On PE: few findings
X-ray: lobar consolidation, + air bronchograms, pleural effusion, occasionally necrosis and cavitation	X-ray: patchy infiltrates
Legionella pneumonia has features of both typical and atypical pneumonia: fever, consolidation, pleural effusion, hyponatremia, GI symptoms	

"Typical" Pneumonias

🔹 The term "typical" in the context of pneumonia implies a bacterial etiology. Lobar consolidation and pleuritic chest pain are characteristics.

🔹 Pneumococcal pneumonia, caused by the pneumococcus (*Streptococcus pneumoniae*) is the prototype of the "typical" pneumonia.

It classically begins with a single shaking chill, cough, pleuritic chest pain, and a steady high fever (not spiking, absent antipyretics). The sputum is typically blood tinged or "rusty." Physical examination reveals signs of consolidation: dullness, increased fremitus, rales, and bronchial breath sounds over the affected area. On chest x-ray lobar consolidation with air bronchograms is the usual finding. A reactive pleural effusion may be present; if so, empyema must be ruled out. Examination of the sputum reveals many polys with intracellular diplococci. Blood cultures may be positive. Strangely, sputum culture fails to grow pneumococci in up to half the cases, for reasons that remain obscure.

🔹 Metastatic infection, although an uncommon complication of pneumococcal pneumonia, is severe and may be life threatening; these sites include the meninges, the aortic valve, and the joints.

🔹 There is a peculiar predilection for pneumococci to infect the sternoclavicular and acromioclavicular joints.

Shoulder pain in a patient with pneumococcal pneumonia or pneumococcal meningitis should prompt evaluation of these joints.

🔹 Some pneumococcal serotypes produce necrotizing lesions in the lung with prominent hemoptysis.

🔹 The pathogenesis of pneumococcal pneumonia requires invasion of the lower respiratory tree.

Since substantial numbers of normal people harbor pneumococci in the nasopharynx without getting sick, particularly in the winter months in temperate climes, a predisposing factor usually can be identified. Pulmonary defense mechanisms are usually adequate to block access to the lower tract; invasion of the alveolar spaces and pneumonia develop when those defense mechanisms are compromised.

🔹 The usual cause of predisposing altered pulmonary defense is a prior viral upper respiratory infection, but other factors that lead to the development of pneumonia include smoking, alcohol intake, stupor, or coma.

Response of pneumococcal pneumonia to penicillin is usually prompt (within a few days). A secondary fever spike may occur as the patient improves 2 to 3 days after the fever breaks; this may reflect cleaning up of the consolidation by the host defenses.

- *Haemophilus influenzae* is another cause of typical pneumonia. The sputum may be "apple green" rather than rusty.

- Staphylococcal pneumonia is a significant cause of postinfluenza morbidity.

A patchy bronchopneumonia with a tendency to cause necrosis and cavitation staph pneumonia requires prompt antibiotic treatment.

- *Klebsiella* pneumonia is a severe gram-negative infection most commonly nosocomial and usually affecting patients with impaired host defense mechanisms such as alcoholism and diabetes. X-ray shows patchy broncopneumonic consolidation frequently with pleural effusions.

- Legionella pneumonia, although bacterial, has many atypical features and should be considered particularly if hyponatremia is prominent and GI symptoms and headache are present (Table 10-1).

Diagnosis of legionella is by urinary antigen or, less useful, direct fluorescent antibody (DFA) testing. Both are specific but lack sensitivity.

Influenza

- Influenza, because of its aggressive attack on the tracheal and bronchial mucosa, is the prototypic predisposition to bacterial pneumonia and bacterial pneumonia is frequently the cause of death in influenza epidemics.

- Although pneumococci are the most frequent cause of pneumonia post influenza, the incidence of staphylococcal pneumonia post influenza is significantly increased.

The latter is a serious infection and delay in treatment of as little as 12 hours may mean the difference between uneventful recovery and extensive lung involvement with necrosis and respiratory failure. Staph pneumonia is usually a patchy bronchopneumonia rather than a dense lobar consolidation.

- Influenza pneumonia, caused by the virus itself rather than bacterial superinfection, is a serious interstitial pneumonitis that may cause severe hypoxemia and death.

The infiltrate may be widespread and cough is productive of a watery serosanguinous, rather than a purulent, sputum.

- Shaking chills and muscle aches are common in influenza and may result in rhabdomyolysis if severe.

CPK may be elevated in severe influenza.

Atypical Pneumonia

Mycoplasma pneumonia is the prototype of the atypical pneumonias; additional etiologic agents include chlamydia, adenovirus, and other respiratory viruses. These infections usually have nonproductive cough, an x-ray picture of patchy nonsegmental infiltrates out of proportion to the clinical examination, which usually reveals a paucity of findings.

> **Pleuritis and pleural effusions are absent** in atypical pneumonias. **Shortness of breath, fatigue, and particularly** headache are commonly associated.

Eosinophilia and Pulmonary Infiltrates

> Chronic eosinophilic pneumonia is a relapsing acute pneumonitis affecting middle-aged women predominately, and characterized by eosinophilic infiltration of the peripheral portions of the lungs.

CBC frequently shows eosinophilia and a past history of asthma is common. Steroid treatment is usually beneficial at inducing remission.

> Eosinophilia in association with pulmonary infiltrates also suggests a drug reaction or Churg–Strauss vasculitis.

SARCOIDOSIS

An immunologic response to as yet unidentified antigens, sarcoidosis is a generalized disease with most prominent involvement in the lung (Table 10-2).

Pulmonary Involvement in Sarcoidosis

> Lung involvement is present in over 90% of patients with sarcoidosis.

The characteristic pathologic findings are scads of noncaseating granulomata with multinucleate giant cells, which are commonly seen on transbronchial biopsy and therefore very useful in establishing the diagnosis.

> The chest x-ray findings in sarcoid include, most prominently, bilateral hilar adenopathy, paratracheal adenopathy, and varying degrees of pulmonary fibrosis depending on the stage.

In advanced stage pulmonary disease, hilar adenopathy disappears and fibrosis dominates the clinical picture. In the United States sarcoidosis is most common in African Americans, particularly women.

Extrapulmonary Manifestations of Sarcoidosis

> Multisystem involvement in sarcoidosis is common.

Extrapulmonary manifestations of sarcoidosis are legion and may include the eye, the pituitary and hypothalamus, peripheral nerves, skin, joints, liver, spleen, lymph nodes, parotid gland, hypercalcemia and hypercalciuria, fever, hypergammaglobulinemia, and cutaneous anergy. The related clinical features may include uveitis, diabetes insipidus, endocrine abnormalities, polyneuritis,

TABLE 10.2 Sarcoidosis

Pathology: noncaseating granulomata in multiple organ systems
Pulmonary involvement (>90%)
Hilar and paratracheal adenopathy
May progress to pulmonary fibrosis
Extrapulmonary features
Cutaneous anergy (negative Tuberculin test)
Uveitis
Polyneuropathy, cranial nerve paresis (facial), CNS, hypothalamus-pituitary
↑ IgG
Hepatomegaly, splenomegaly, lymphadenopathy
Arthritis
Skin (papules, plaques, erythema nodosum, lupus pernio)
Hypercalciuria
Fever
Acute presentations
Lofgren's syndrome (hilar adenopathy, arthritis, erythema nodosum, fever)
Heerfordt's syndrome (hilar adenopathy, parotid and lacrimal swelling, fever)

and cranial nerve palsies (principally the VII – Bell's palsy), splenomegaly, and lymphadenopathy. Hepatic involvement with granulomas is common but usually subclinical, although the alkaline phosphatase may be elevated.

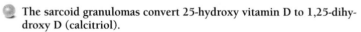 **The tuberculin test is always negative in sarcoidosis.**

The sarcoid granulomas convert 25-hydroxy vitamin D to 1,25-dihydroxy D (calcitriol).

The unregulated production of the active form of vitamin D increases calcium absorption from the gut and rarely (5% to 10%) causes hypercalcemia, but commonly (50%) causes hypercalciuria. Granulomas in other diseases such as lymphomas and tuberculosis may synthesize calcitriol as well, but less commonly than in sarcoidosis.

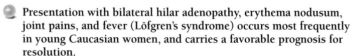 **Presentation with bilateral hilar adenopathy, erythema nodosum, joint pains, and fever (Löfgren's syndrome) occurs most frequently in young Caucasian women, and carries a favorable prognosis for resolution.**

Other skin manifestations include a dramatic swelling of the soft tissues of the nose with reddish plaques (lupus pernio) and nonspecific papulosquamous lesions frequently associated with arthritis. Lupus pernio presages a poor long-term prognosis.

⚫ **Acute presentation of sarcoid with parotid and lacrimal gland swelling and fever, in addition to hilar adenopathy, is known as Heerfordt's syndrome.**

TUBERCULOSIS (TB)
Upper Lobe Localization
⚫ **After primary infection (Ghon complex – typical mid lung field, subpleural lesion with associated hilar adenopathy) TB localizes in the apex of the lung (posterior segment of the upper lobe) where it remains, alive but quiescent, and serves as a nidus for reactivation.**

Localization in the upper lobe, where oxygen is at its highest concentration, reflects the microaerophilic predilection of *Mycobacterium tuberculosis*. The "tuberculous habitus" has been referred to as tall and thin since the days of Hippocrates, possibly for the same reason (better aerated upper lobes), although the significance of this association in the pathogenesis of TB has been called into question.

⚫ **Volume loss in the upper lobe due to scarring and fibrosis is the typical radiographic finding of chronic pulmonary TB.**

Reactivation of latent TB may occur at any subsequent time but immunosuppression from any cause, particularly treatment with corticosteroids or antibodies to tumor necrosis factor (TNF), is an important antecedent of reactivation.

⚫ **Bronchiectasis involving the upper lobes should raise the suspicion of TB.**

Other possible causes of upper lobe bronchiectasis include postinfluenza, cystic fibrosis, sarcoidosis, and allergic bronchopulmonary aspergillosis (ABPA).

Pleural Effusions with TB
⚫ **Tuberculous pleural effusions, classically an extrapulmonary manifestation following primary TB infection, is exudative, lymphocytic, small to moderate in size, unilateral, and associated with fever, cough, and pleuritic chest pain.**

In effusions complicating primary infection the chest x-ray is negative except for the pleural fluid. The pathogenesis involves rupture of a subpleural caseous lesion with spillage into the pleural space; the resulting exudative effusion is thought to represent hypersensitivity to tubercular proteins.

- The tuberculin skin test is always positive in cases of tuberculous pleurisy with effusion (absent a state of cutaneous anergy).

- Smear of the pleural fluid is almost always negative and culture is positive in about one-half of the cases. Pleural biopsy (histology demonstrating granulomas plus organisms and culture) is the time-honored method of diagnosis.

- Although tuberculous effusions resolve spontaneously, recognition of the effusion as a manifestation of primary TB is important since untreated there is a high incidence of pulmonary and extrapulmonary TB developing within months or years.

- Tuberculous effusions may also complicate reactivation TB.

In these cases parenchymal disease is usually obvious.

Extrathoracic Tuberculosis

- Extrapulmonary complications of TB frequently occur in the absence of obvious pulmonary disease.

Hematogenous dissemination of the *tubercle bacillus* may cause disease at many sites including bones and joints, meninges, vertebrae and epidural space (Pott's disease), psoas muscle, breast (mimics cancer), pericardium, and, most commonly, the genitourinary system.

- Sterile pyuria is the classic manifestation of genitourinary (GU) tuberculosis, and hematuria, which may be severe, is very common, reflecting extensive involvement of the renal pelvis and collecting system.

Acid fast stain of the urine is frequently positive. Calcification of the epididymis in men is a frequent manifestation of genitourinary TB, and is particularly common in patients from Haiti.

- Hematogenous TB may infect the liver as well in the severe septicemic form of the disease.

TB in the liver carries the colorful eponym "the typhobacillosis of Landouzy."

ASPERGILLOSIS

- Aspergillosis affects the lung in three ways: ABPA, fungus ball (aspergilloma), and invasive aspergillus pneumonia.

- ABPA is a hypersensitivity reaction to Aspergillus antigens that produces wheezing, cough, and brownish sputum.

ABPA occurs in patients with pre-existing asthma or, less commonly, cystic fibrosis, and is characterized by very high IgE levels and positive tests for allergy to *Aspergillus*. Fleeting infiltrates (frequently upper lobe) on chest x-ray and peripheral eosinophilia are common. Upper lobe bronchiectasis may develop as well. The acute phase responds well to prednisone; antifungal treatment may be required for refractory disease.

- **Aspergilloma is a clump of fungus (mycetoma) that occurs in a pre-existing cavity and is usually an incidental finding although it may invade the cavity wall and cause significant hemoptysis.**

- **Invasive Aspergillus pneumonia is a disease of immunocompromised patients. It frequently occurs in neutropenic patients receiving chemotherapy.**

It has a predilection to invade the pulmonary arterial tree causing lung infarction and necrotizing pneumonia.

- **Immunocompetent patients with pneumonia who grow Aspergillus in the sputum after antibiotic treatment do not have invasive Aspergillus pneumonia.**

In this situation the *Aspergillus* is a nonpathogenic saprophyte.

PULMONARY THROMBOEMBOLIC DISEASE

- **Pulmonary embolus (PE) and pulmonary infarction are not synonymous.**

- **An embolus to the pulmonary vasculature produces symptoms that depend on the size of the embolus and the extent of the pulmonary vasculature that is occluded.**

A PE may be asymptomatic, may cause dyspnea, and, if large enough, may cause right heart strain and shock.

- **Pulmonary infarction is necrosis of lung tissue that involves the parietal pleura, is always symptomatic with pleuritis, and usually associated with a small pleural effusion.**

Infarction follows embolization when the midsize arteries are occluded and particularly when the pulmonary circulation is compromised usually as a result of CHF. In addition to the CT angiogram, lung scan and cardiac echo are important diagnostic modalities in assessing pulmonary embolization.

- **A completely normal lung scan rules out PE. In the evaluation of shock a dilated right ventricle points to pulmonary embolization as the underlying cause.**

- **Chronic venous thromboembolism (VTE) is an important cause of pulmonary hypertension and needs to be distinguished from primary pulmonary hypertension.**

The distinction is not always easy. Primary pulmonary hypertension is most common in young women. Chronic VTE may be distinguished by imaging techniques that show fresh or organized pulmonary emboli, but in the presence of significant pulmonary hypertension in situ thrombosis may occur rendering the distinction difficult.

 Chronic pulmonary hypertension results in atherosclerosis of the pulmonary arterial tree (Ayerza's disease) which predisposes to in situ thrombosis.

Atherosclerotic thrombosis in the pulmonary arteries is difficult, if not impossible, to distinguish from embolic disease; anticoagulation is indicated in both conditions.

The Gastrointestinal Tract, Pancreas, and Liver

CHAPTER 11

THE GASTROINTESTINAL TRACT

Functional Gastrointestinal Disease

One clinical challenge posed by gastrointestinal (GI) tract symptoms is to distinguish the so-called "functional" (nonpathologic) from the "organic" (structural or pathologic) disorders, since some patients have hyperawareness of normal GI functions that may cause a variety of symptoms.

Psychological factors play a role in some of these functional symptom complexes.

Vomiting before breakfast is virtually always functional; diarrhea that does not disturb sleep at night is unlikely to represent a serious disease.

In evaluating diarrhea the presence of urgency, tenesmus, and fecal incontinence suggest lesions involving the distal sigmoid colon and rectum.

Large volume diarrhea without the above symptoms suggests a small bowel site of involvement.

Irritable Bowel Syndrome

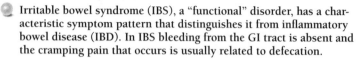 Irritable bowel syndrome (IBS), a "functional" disorder, has a characteristic symptom pattern that distinguishes it from inflammatory bowel disease (IBD). In IBS bleeding from the GI tract is absent and the cramping pain that occurs is usually related to defecation.

Diarrhea is the major symptom but intermittent bouts of constipation occur as well.

The characteristic pattern of the diarrhea in IBS is four or five bowel movements in the morning, ending by noon.

Bleeding or nocturnal diarrhea necessitates a work up for IBD.

Inflammatory Bowel Disease

IBD, Crohn's disease and ulcerative colitis (UC), have some similarities and many distinctions. UC is limited to the colon; Crohn's involves the small bowel, the colon, or both.

Crohn's disease is characterized by abdominal pain and, when the colon is involved, by GI bleeding.

Ineffable fatigue is a particularly debilitating feature of moderate to severe Crohn's disease.

Bleeding is invariable in UC because it is a mucosal disease.

The inflammation in UC progresses contiguously from the rectosigmoid; the inflammation in Crohn's disease involves the ileum and the right colon with many "skip" areas.

The inflammatory process in Crohn's disease is transmural, frequently with granuloma formation, and a tendency to form fistulas. Small bowel involvement in Crohn's disease is a frequent cause of intestinal obstruction.

Small bowel involvement in UC is limited to "backwash" ileitis.

UC is cured by colectomy; surgical resection in Crohn's disease usually results in the re-emergence of Crohn's disease in the unresected previously normal bowel.

Pancolitis in long-standing UC is associated with a high incidence of carcinoma, a fact favoring colectomy. The risk of colon cancer is increased in Crohn's disease, but much less so.

Extraintestinal manifestations are common in IBD. These presumably have an immunologic basis, and include arthritis; erythema nodosum; episcleritis and uveitis; and with Crohn's disease, mucosal erosions.

The systemic manifestations in Crohn's disease (fever, fatigue, anemia, and elevated indicia of inflammation) respond well to antagonists of tumor necrosis factor.

Long-standing inflammation in patients with Crohn's disease may result in secondary amyloidosis (AA).

Crohn's disease is occasionally misdiagnosed as Behcet's disease in patients who present with fever, arthritis, iritis or episcleritis, and mucosal ulcerations.

The bowel symptoms in patients with Crohn's disease may appear well after the above mentioned manifestations thereby causing confusion. In patients from the United States, not of Middle Eastern descent, Crohn's disease, and not Behcet's disease, is the usual diagnosis.

The arthritis associated with IBD (enteropathic arthritis) may involve the hips, knees, and the small joints of the hand.

Deformities and bony erosions are very uncommon. An immunologic basis is presumed and activity of the joint disease frequently occurs with flares of the bowel disease.

Sacroiliac or spinal involvement (spondyloarthropathy) also occurs with IBD and is frequently associated with the HLA-B27 histocompatibility antigen.

The spondyloarthropathy may antedate the onset of bowel disease by several years.

Gastrointestinal Bleeding from Peptic Ulcer Disease

Upper GI bleeding (rostral to the ligament of Trietz) is much more common than bleeding from a lower GI site. Peptic ulcer remains the most common cause of UGI bleeding followed in frequency by esophageal or gastric varices secondary to portal hypertension.

The identification of *Helicobacter pylori* as an important cause of peptic ulcer disease and the development of effective strategies for eradicating the organism, along with the development of potent proton pump inhibitors, has decreased the prevalence of peptic ulcer and its complications. Nonetheless, peptic ulcer is still the most important source of upper GI bleeding.

Epigastric pain that wakes the patient at night is particularly characteristic of peptic ulcer since gastric acid secretion is at its peak at about 2 AM.

Peptic ulcer never causes pain on awakening in the morning since gastric acid secretion is at its low point at this time.

Many patients who present with upper GI bleeding from peptic ulcer will have no symptoms of prior peptic disease.

⚬ The physical signs of acute perforation of a peptic ulcer are striking. In addition to the classic "board-like rigidity" pain at the top of the right shoulder and resonance over the liver are characteristic.

Shoulder pain reflects diaphragmatic irritation and is felt in the distribution of C 3, 4, 5. Hyperresonance over the normally dull liver is particularly striking.

⚬ Elevation of the BUN relative to the creatinine level is a very useful indication of an upper GI bleeding site.

Two factors favor BUN elevation with an upper GI bleed. 1) Diminished blood volume and blood pressure cause renal arterial vasoconstriction and thus decrease renal blood flow more than creatinine clearance. Decreased renal blood flow preferentially diminishes urea clearance because of back diffusion of urea in the distal nephron, a process sensitive to blood flow. 2) The protein load in the small bowel from the digestion of intraluminal blood results in increased urea production. Coupled with the renal hemodynamic changes, an increase in the gut protein load raises the BUN relative to the creatinine.

Hereditary Hemorrhagic Telangiectasia (Osler–Weber–Rendu Disease)

⚬ Hereditary hemorrhagic telangiectasia is a rare but significant cause of GI bleeding. Inherited as an autosomal dominant trait and consisting of telangiectasias (small arteriovenous anastomoses) located principally on mucosal surfaces, the disease usually manifests as GI bleeding in early adult life.

⚬ Telangiectasias on the lips are often visible but frequently overlooked, particularly in anemic patients or those who have just experienced GI bleeding.

They manifest as small red macules that may have a square or rectangular shape and may be slightly raised. It is not uncommon for these to appear clinically after transfusions have been administered (just in time for the attending to make the diagnosis on the morning following admission). Bleeding may be chronic and low grade or brisk. Iron deficiency anemia is commonly present.

⚬ Epistaxis, particularly in childhood, reflects the location of these lesions on the nasal mucosa, and provides an important historical clue to the diagnosis in patients presenting in adulthood with GI bleeding.

Lesions may also occur in the lungs and if sufficiently large may result in a right to left shunt. Rarely lesions in the CNS may cause subarachnoid or brain hemorrhage or brain abscess (strategically placed A-V anastomoses which broach the blood–brain barrier).

Lower Gastrointestinal Bleeding

 Lower gastrointestinal bleeding with a "negative" colonoscopy is either from angiomas (angiodysplasia) or diverticular vessels, since it is frequently difficult to identify bleeding that originates from these sites by endoscopy.

Diverticular bleeding may be heavy but usually stops on its own.

Malabsorption

Malabsorption in adults may be caused by celiac sprue (nontropical sprue), bacterial overgrowth, tropical sprue, pancreatic enzyme deficiency, and certain infections (Table 11-1).

 Steatorrhea, weight loss, diarrhea, and vitamin deficiencies are the major manifestations of malabsorption.

The diagnosis of malabsorption is confirmed by demonstrating fat in the stools, which are usually greasy, bulky, and foul smelling.

TABLE 11.1 Malabsorption

Disease	Etiology	Diagnosis	Treatment
Celiac sprue	Gluten sensitivity	IgA antibodies (anti-tTG, anti-EMA) small bowel biopsy	Gluten-free diet
Tropical sprue	Infection + folate deficiency	Clinical + endemic area exposure	Antibiotics + folate
Bacterial over-growth	Bile salt deconjugation from surgical blind loop, small bowel diverticulae, stasis from bowel infiltration or dysmotility	History + GI tract imaging	Antibiotics
Pancreatic in-sufficiency	Chronic pancreatitis, surgery	History, chronic alcoholism	Oral pancreatic enzymes
Zollinger–Ellison syndrome	Hyperacidity inactivates pancreatic lipase	Peptic ulcer disease hyperacidity	Proton pump inhibitors (PPIs), surgery

🔵 Vitamin deficiencies are characteristic manifestations of malabsorption: fat soluble vitamins are lost in fecal fat; mucosal abnormalities are the cause of folate and B_{12} malabsorption.

The associated clinical picture reflects the function of the deficient vitamin.

🔵 Severe vitamin D deficiency is associated with rickets in children and osteomalacia in adults. The alkaline phosphatase level (from osteoblasts) is always elevated and provides a useful guide to treatment with vitamin D.

Normalization of the alkaline phosphatase reflects adequate treatment with vitamin D.

Celiac Disease

🔵 Celiac sprue (also known as celiac disease, gluten enteropathy, or nontropical sprue), caused by sensitivity to the wheat protein gluten, may be clinically manifest for the first time in adults of any age.

🔵 Although the manifestations of celiac disease may be subtle iron and folate deficiency are commonly present.

Iron and folate absorption are impaired in celiac disease since they are absorbed in the proximal small bowel, the region where the mucosal abnormality in sprue is the greatest.

🔵 Shorter than expected stature is a useful clue to the diagnosis of celiac disease in adulthood.

Comparison of the height of the patient with that of the parents and siblings may serve as a reference point for short stature. Presumably, nutritional deficiency, even in the absence of characteristic symptoms of malabsorption, is the cause.

🔵 Celiac disease is diagnosed by serologic tests, small intestinal biopsy, and the response to a gluten-free diet.

🔵 IgA antibodies directed at tissue transglutaminase (tTG-IgA) and endomysial antibodies (EMA-IgA) have high specificity and sensitivity for celiac sprue, the former being the currently preferred initial test.

Small bowel biopsy is confirmatory showing a characteristic picture of flattened, atrophic villi and lymphocytic infiltration. The clinical manifestations and the histologic abnormalities are corrected on a gluten-free diet.

🔵 Intestinal lymphoma is an uncommon but troublesome complication of celiac sprue.

🔵 Celiac disease is associated with the unique (and rare) dermatologic disease known as dermatitis herpetiformis (DH) since it consists of crops of vesicles.

Most patients with DH have at least some evidence of celiac disease, but most patients with celiac disease do not have DH.

🔵 **Many patients who do not have sprue report "sensitivity" to gluten.**

These patients feel better on gluten-free diets for reasons not understood. This "sensitivity" has been addressed by the food industry with a proliferation of gluten-free foods.

Tropical Sprue

🔵 **Tropical sprue, in distinction to celiac disease (nontropical sprue), is a malabsorption syndrome endemic in tropical regions, and is probably caused by a combination of bacterial infection and vitamin deficiency, particularly that of folic acid.**

Endemic in the tropics, particularly the Caribbean, Southeast Asia, and southern India, nontropical sprue also affects visitors on prolonged stays in these regions. Onset is frequently with fever and diarrhea followed by chronic diarrhea and malabsorption.

🔵 **Megaloblastic anemia is common in tropical sprue because of the folic acid deficiency and, occasionally, an associated B_{12} deficiency, the latter because folate deficiency affects the ileal mucosa and impairs B_{12} absorption.**

Treatment entails a long course of antibiotics and folate.

Bacterial Overgrowth

🔵 **Bacterial overgrowth in the small bowel may occur when motility is disturbed from autonomic neuropathy or an infiltrative process, when a blind loop is created surgically, in the presence of a large diverticulum in the duodenum or jejunum, or when a fistula connects the colon with the small intestine.**

Ordinarily, the small bowel contains only a fraction of the bacteria found in the colon; an increase in the small bowel population of bacteria affects the mucosa and alters the metabolism of bile salts.

🔵 **Steatorrhea occurs with bacterial overgrowth because the bacteria deconjugate bile salts, thereby affecting the micelles that are essential for normal fat absorption.**

🔵 **Diarrhea complicates bacterial overgrowth since unconjugated bile acids irritate the colonic mucosa.**

🔵 **B_{12} deficiency may occur with bacterial overgrowth since the bacteria compete with the host for cyanocobalamin; folate does not become deficient in overgrowth situations since the overgrown bacteria produce folate.**

Treatment entails surgical correction of the abnormality where possible; broad-spectrum antibiotics when the abnormality responsible for the overgrowth cannot be fixed as in diabetic neuropathy, scleroderma, or amyloid infiltration.

Pancreatic Insufficiency

Destruction of the pancreatic acinar tissue in chronic alcoholic pancreatitis, or inactivation of pancreatic lipase by hyperacidity in the presence of a gastrinoma, are the usual pancreatic causes of malabsorption.

Pancreatic enzymes supplied orally, and treatment of gastric hyperacidity, constitute treatment which is generally effective.

Infections and Malabsorption

Two infections may be associated with significant malabsorption: Whipple's disease and giardiasis.

Whipple's disease, a widespread indolent infection with the gram-positive, PAS-positive, bacterium *Tropheryma whipplei*, infects the small intestine along with many other organs.

Malabsorption occurs late in the course of the disease which has a predilection for middle-aged white men and is associated with arthritis as an early manifestation. Intestinal biopsy demonstrating scads of PAS-positive macrophages establishes the diagnosis.

Giardiasis, caused by the protozoal parasite *Giardia lamblia,* has a worldwide distribution and is spread by cysts that survive in cold water and by fecal–oral person-to-person transmission.

Campers may be infected from cold water streams, and day care attendees from poor fecal hygiene. Water-borne epidemics also occur. The infection is not invasive but may cause an acute gastroenteritis; many cases are asymptomatic. In a minority of cases a prolonged chronic illness develops and in these cases malabsorption with weight loss may be prominent.

Zollinger–Ellison Syndrome (Gastrinoma)

Hyperacidity in the duodenum from gastric hypersecretion may inactivate pancreatic lipase giving rise to malabsorption.

THE PANCREAS

Acute Pancreatitis

Acute pancreatitis has several causes: alcohol, gall stones, hypertriglyceridemia, many drugs, instrumentation of the biliary ducts, and congenital anatomic abnormalities of the pancreatic ducts.

By far the most common causes are alcohol and gall stones. The common denominator of all the causes is autodigestion of the gland by the pancreatic enzymes which are released and activated by increased pressure in the obstructed pancreatic duct and by the cellular injury and duodenal inflammation induced by alcohol. The diagnosis is established by elevated plasma levels of amylase and lipase in the right clinical setting. The lipase level is more specific since amylase is produced by other tissues and amylase levels are elevated in other diseases as well as pancreatitis.

- **Epigastric pain radiating to the back with vomiting is the classic (and usual) presentation. Vomiting is almost invariable in all but the mildest of cases. Nothing by mouth is tolerated. Even sips of water cause reflex retching.**

A common mistake in treating acute pancreatitis is feeding too quickly. Oral feeding stimulates pancreatic secretion which prolongs the inflammation. Once the pain subsides refeeding can begin.

- **It makes absolutely no sense to begin feeding patients with acute pancreatitis who still require narcotics for pain.**

- **In severe cases of pancreatitis extensive exudation in the abdomen occurs with local fat necrosis and the sequestration of large amounts of fluid.**

The hematocrit may be very high (60%) due to hemoconcentration. Large amounts of fluid may be required early in the course of treatment to maintain the adequacy of the circulation.

- **Seepage of blood from the inflamed pancreas into the umbilicus or the flanks gives rise to Cullen's and Grey–Turner's signs respectively.**

- **Left-sided pleural effusion may also occur with pleuritis and atelectasis of the left lower lobe.**

- **Fat necrosis in acute pancreatitis may occur inside or outside the abdomen due to circulating pancreatic lipases; hydrolysis of triglycerides into free fatty acids then ensues, followed by saponification with calcium, resulting, in severe cases, in hypocalcemia.**

The latter is a poor prognostic sign. It is no surprise that pancreatic inflammation may also impair insulin secretion giving rise to hyperglycemia.

- **Many years of heavy drinking usually precede the initial attack of pancreatitis. Recurrent bouts are the rule especially if the drinking continues.**

In alcoholic pancreatitis damage to the pancreas is well established before the first acute attack occurs.

- **Stones in the biliary tract that obstruct the pancreatic duct are the other major cause of acute pancreatitis.**

Passing a common duct stone may cause acute pancreatitis that varies in severity from mild to very severe. The amylase and lipase levels may be very high since the pancreas in these cases was normal prior to the passage of the stone. The enzyme elevations in this situation do not reflect the severity of the pancreatitis.

- Hypertriglyceridemia is an uncommon but well recognized cause of acute pancreatitis. The triglyceride level is usually above 1,000 mg/dL in affected patients and the blood appears "milky" or lactescent.

- Lipemia retinalis is frequently noted on presentation in patients with triglyceride induced pancreatitis. Eruptive xanthomas may be present as well.

The blood in the vessels of the optic fundus looks like "cream of tomato" soup. Eruptive xanthomas are small yellow papules often with an erythematous base that may appear anywhere but are particularly common on the buttocks.

- High triglyceride levels may obscure the diagnosis of pancreatitis by interfering with the amylase determination rendering it falsely low.

Lipase levels are probably not affected.

- The elevated triglycerides usually reflect an impairment in lipoprotein lipase so that chylomicrons or chylomicrons plus very low density lipoprotein (VLDL) triglycerides are elevated (type I and type V in the Fredrickson classification of hyperlipidemias).

Frequently congenital, the defect in lipoprotein lipase may be induced by drugs such as alcohol or estrogen, or may occur *de novo* in pregnancy.

- Hypertriglyceridemia is the most common cause of pancreatitis developing in pregnancy.

The high estrogen levels are the presumed cause.

- Pancreatic divisum, a congenital anomaly in which the embryonic dorsal and ventral pancreatic ducts fail to fuse, is an uncommon cause of acute and chronic pancreatitis.

Although most people with this anomaly are asymptomatic, in young patients without a history of alcoholism or gall stones the possibility of pancreatic divisum should be considered. Imaging the ducts establishes the diagnosis and sphincterotomy may be useful in treating recurrent attacks.

- Drug-induced pancreatitis is a particular problem in HIV patients who take Bactrim for prophylaxis of pneumocystis pneumonia (PCP) as well as antiviral agents.

BILIARY TRACT DISEASE

In addition to causing pancreatitis gall stones may cause biliary colic and acute cholecystitis (Table 11-2).

TABLE 11.2 Biliary Tract Diseases

Biliary colic	
Stone in the cystic duct. Waxing and waning RUQ pain; cannot lie still	
Acute cholecystitis	
Impacted stone in cystic duct→ acute inflammation with fever, RUQ tenderness, vomiting	
Common duct stone	
Biliary obstruction with jaundice and high risk of pancreatitis	
Ascending cholangitis	
Infection of the biliary tree with gut flora. Progressive jaundice, fever, sepsis	
Primary sclerosing cholangitis	
Sclerosis of bile ducts; unknown cause; male predominance; highly (80%) associated with ulcerative colitis; negative anti-mitochondrial antibody (AMA)	
Secondary sclerosing cholangitis	
Sclerosis of bile ducts following obstruction and infection from stones, strictures, or cancer	
Primary biliary cirrhosis	
Autoimmune disease of middle aged women; + AMA; ↑ alkaline phosphatase, ↑ bilirubin; intense pruritus; hypertriglyceridemia	
Secondary biliary cirrhosis	
Long-standing biliary tract obstruction; digital clubbing common; negative AMA	
Cholangiocarcinoma	
Adenocarcinoma of the biliary epithelium; associated with biliary obstruction; when located at the bifurcation of the biliary ducts known as "Klatskin tumor"	

Biliary Colic and Acute Cholecystitis

Biliary colic is the waxing and waning right upper quadrant pain caused by a stone in the cystic duct. If the stone becomes impacted acute cholecystitis develops with associated fever, chills, and vomiting.

The pain of acute cholecystitis is inflammatory in nature (made worse by movement and deep inspiration). It may radiate to the back or the top of the right shoulder if the diaphragm is contiguous to the inflammation. It is distinguishable from the pain of biliary colic which is associated with writhing around as the pain comes and goes.

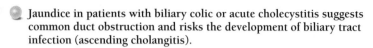 Jaundice in patients with biliary colic or acute cholecystitis suggests common duct obstruction and risks the development of biliary tract infection (ascending cholangitis).

Cholestasis refers to obstruction to the normal flow of bile from the liver. Biliary tract obstruction may be intrahepatic (hepatitis), extrahepatic, or both. There are many different causes including stones, strictures, tumors, and autoimmunity. Elevation of alkaline phosphatase is the earliest liver function test affected.

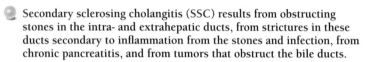 Secondary sclerosing cholangitis (SSC) results from obstructing stones in the intra- and extrahepatic ducts, from strictures in these ducts secondary to inflammation from the stones and infection, from chronic pancreatitis, and from tumors that obstruct the bile ducts.

 Primary sclerosing cholangitis (PSC) is scarring and narrowing of the extra- and intrahepatic bile ducts in the absence of the factors listed above that cause SSC.

Both PSC and SSC are associated with an increased risk of cholangiocarcinoma.

 PSC is closely related to ulcerative colitis (UC) which is associated with PSC in at least 80% of cases. The disease is most common in young to middle-aged men.

The pathogenesis of PSC is unknown although a number of associations suggest that genetic, immunologic, and perhaps infectious, agents predispose to the disease. Thus, HLA type, p-ANCA, and even IgG4-related disease have been associated in some cases. Portal bacteremia from breakdown in the mucosal barrier in UC has been implicated as well. Antimitochondrial antibodies, a hallmark of primary biliary cirrhosis (PBC), are absent.

Biliary Cirrhosis

 The consequence of chronic biliary tract obstruction, regardless of the cause, is biliary cirrhosis.

Inflammation in the portal triads is followed by bile duct reduplication, bile staining, hepatocyte necrosis, regenerating nodules, and eventually cirrhosis with portal hypertension and hepatic failure.

 Secondary biliary cirrhosis follows long-standing bile duct obstruction.

 Primary biliary cirrhosis (PBC) is an autoimmune disease of middle-aged women (in distinction to PSC which affects predominantly men). Antimitochondrial antibodies are sensitive and specific for this diagnosis. The alkaline phosphatase is elevated. Intense pruritus and fatigue are early symptoms.

The autoimmune attack is directed at the biliary epithelium of the small intrahepatic bile ducts which results in inflammation, scarring, and obliteration of the ducts.

Bile acid binding resins (cholestyramine) may ameliorate the itching.

- Biliary cirrhosis is associated with a characteristic lipid abnormality in which intermediate density lipoproteins (IDLs) are elevated as well as high density lipoproteins (HDLs) (type III hyperlipidemia in the Fredrickson classification). This is associated with unique palmar and palmar crease xanthomas, but not with an increased risk of cardiovascular disease.

- Digital clubbing may also be associated with biliary cirrhosis.

Although all forms of cirrhosis may be associated with clubbing the latter is most common in the biliary form of the disease.

PORTAL CIRRHOSIS

- Cirrhosis is the final common pathway of liver damage from a variety of causes that result in necrosis of hepatocytes, collapse of the normal liver architecture, nodular regeneration, and destruction of the normal portal venous system with the development of portal hypertension.

The top causes of portal, as compared with biliary cirrhosis considered above, are the viral hepatitides (posthepatitic cirrhosis), excessive alcohol intake (Laennec's cirrhosis), and fatty infiltration (nonalcoholic steatohepatitis [NASH]); less common causes include chronic passive congestion (cardiac cirrhosis from long-standing CHF) and inherited metabolic abnormalities including hemochromatosis, Wilson's disease, and alpha-1 antitrypsin deficiency.

- Cirrhosis of any kind predisposes to hepatocellular carcinoma (HCC).

- Elevated levels of alpha-fetoprotein (AFP) suggest the development of HCC and are useful for monitoring therapy since in patients with HCC these levels correlate with tumor size.

The chronic inflammation and regeneration of the liver appears to be the major mechanism of malignant transformation in cirrhosis, but with viral etiologies a direct effect of the viral genome may be involved.

- The physical stigmata of cirrhosis reflect portal hypertension and, in men, hypogonadism with low testosterone and high estrogens.

Ascites, splenomegaly, increased abdominal venous pattern, caput medusa reflect portal hypertension; gynecomastia, testicular atrophy, loss of axillary hair, spider angiomata, and palmar erythema reflect principally the high estrogen to testosterone ratio (hypogonadism).

- Parotid and lacrimal gland hypertrophy also occur in cirrhotics for reasons that remain obscure.

Alcoholism and malnutrition may be involved. Osteoporosis is common as well.

🔹 The major complications related to portal hypertension are ascites (sometimes massive), variceal bleeding (sometimes massive), hypersplenism, hepatic encephalopathy, spontaneous bacterial peritonitis (SBP), and hepatorenal syndrome.

Variceal hemorrhage is a relatively common cause of upper GI bleeding. Bleeding from varices is usually brisk, although small bleeds are not uncommon.

🔹 In a patient with gastroesophageal varices a small bleed frequently heralds the onset of a major hematemesis.

This "herald" bleed serves as a warning that urgent treatment of the varices is needed.

The ascites that occurs with portal hypertension is transudative and contains few cells, mostly lymphocytes, unless complicated by SBP.

🔹 SBP is caused by enteric organisms that traverse the congested intestinal mucosal barrier and directly infect the ascetic fluid.

🔹 SBP should be suspected in any decompensated cirrhotic patient with significant ascites. Fever and abdominal findings are typically absent in SBP, although abdominal discomfort may be present. The diagnosis is made by the presence of polymorphonuclear leukocytes in ascitic fluid obtained from a diagnostic paracentesis.

🔹 A diagnostic paracentesis should be performed on all cirrhotics presenting in a decompensated state to rule out SBP.

A total cell count of $100/\mu L$ with over 50% polys is highly suggestive and warrants treatment. The smear is always negative and the culture frequently unrevealing.

🔹 In patients with massive ascites large volume paracentesis may be required for comfort's sake but carries significant downside risk including infection, protein depletion, and the possibility of inducing variceal hemorrhage.

The latter may occur by altering interabdominal hemodynamics. Releasing the tamponade induced by tense ascites may increase portal blood flow and decrease the external pressure on varices, thereby increasing flow through the varices leading to rupture.

On the positive side paracentesis in conjunction with plasma volume support may help initiate a diuresis by relieving pressure on the renal veins and increasing renal blood flow.

Hepatic Encephalopathy

🔹 Hepatic encephalopathy, a serious complication of cirrhosis, is a consequence of portal hypertension which shunts blood from the portal to the systemic circulation, thereby eliminating the hepatic detoxification of nitrogenous compounds from the gut (Table 11-3).

TABLE 11.3 Hepatic Encephalopathy

Cause: portal hypertension

Nitrogenous compounds from bacterial metabolism of protein in the gut bypass detoxification in the liver

Metabolic encephalopathy:

Drowsiness, lethargy, stupor, coma (rarely, agitation, violent behavior)

Asterixis

Respiratory alkalosis

Hyperreflexia, clonus, opisthotonos

Precipitating causes

↑ dietary protein

GI bleeding

Constipation

Alkalosis

Sedative medications

Treatment

Lactulose → diarrhea, acidifies stool

Nonabsorbable antibiotics → decrease bacterial metabolism of protein

---

Mild cognitive impairment is at one end of the spectrum of hepatic encephalopathy, life-threatening coma is at the other end.

- Although drowsiness, lethargy, and stupor are most common, some patients present with agitation and bizarre behavior.

- The pathogenesis of hepatic encephalopathy is uncertain but nitrogenous compounds formed in the gut are almost certainly involved. Ammonia levels are usually elevated but do not correlate with the severity of the encephalopathy. Ammonia may be a marker for an array of other amines that escape metabolism in the liver.

In severe cases increased intracranial pressure supervenes. EEG shows the triphasic waves characteristic of metabolic encephalopathy, but is not specific for hepatic encephalopathy.

- Asterixis is the most common physical finding, and although highly characteristic of hepatic encephalopathy, it also occurs in other metabolic encephalopathies. In the setting of chronic liver disease however, asterixis is virtually diagnostic of hepatic encephalopathy.

Asterixis, the inability to hold a position, is tested by extending the hands at the wrist joints ("stopping traffic"). The "flap" that results is a positive test.

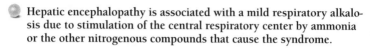 Hepatic encephalopathy is associated with a mild respiratory alkalosis due to stimulation of the central respiratory center by ammonia or the other nitrogenous compounds that cause the syndrome.

All of the acid–base problems that complicate decompensated cirrhosis occur in the setting of this baseline respiratory alkalosis.

 Hyperreflexia is almost invariable with hepatic encephalopathy and may be severe with clonus and, in some cases, opisthotonos.

 The coma of hepatic encephalopathy may be profound. It represents the deepest coma from which virtually complete recovery is possible.

Be very reluctant to pronounce a patient with hepatic encephalopathy "brain dead."

 In patients with portal hypertension the precipitating causes of hepatic encephalopathy include GI bleeding, constipation, alkalosis, volume depletion, sedative medications, intercurrent infections (particularly SBP), and dietary protein excess.

Blood in the gut and increased protein ingestion ("one meatball syndrome") provide substrate for intestinal bacteria to generate the nitrogenous compounds that escape detoxification. Constipation increases the absorption of these compounds.

Alkalosis favors the formation of the freely diffusible form of ammonia (NH_3) and other amines over the cationic ammonium (NH_4) ion. The NH3 and free amines penetrate the CNS well while the ammonium form is excluded.

Volume depletion stimulates aldosterone which results in hypokalemic alkalosis.

The treatment of hepatic encephalopathy depends on reversing these factors to the extent possible.

 Lactulose causes diarrhea and, most importantly, acidifies the stool as it is metabolized to lactic acid by gut bacteria, thereby decreasing the production of free NH_3. Nonabsorbable antibiotics diminish the intestinal flora that generate the nitrogenous compounds that cause the syndrome.

It goes without saying that avoiding drugs that depress the CNS and treating intercurrent infections are part of the therapeutic regimen.

Hepatorenal Syndrome (HRS) and Hepatopulmonary Syndrome

 Hepatorenal syndrome (HRS), an important complication of decompensated cirrhosis, carries a high mortality rate. Ascites is always present and edema is usual. The kidneys are intrinsically normal; the environment created by decompensated liver failure is the cause, although the precise mechanisms remain unknown.

🔵 HRS is caused by a decrease in renal blood flow that occurs despite the fact that the extracellular fluid volume is expanded. Plasma renin levels are high (attesting to the diminished renal blood flow), and secondary aldosteronism is present. Hypoalbuminemia is present as well from diminished hepatic synthesis.

Hyponatremia results from inability to excrete water normally in the face of diminished renal blood flow. Hypokalemia reflects the secondary aldosteronism as well as diarrhea and poor intake.

🔵 The urinary sodium is low in HRS reflecting poor renal perfusion.

The blood pressure in cirrhotics is typically low and a trial of pressors may be warranted to increase renal blood flow although patients with HRS rarely respond. The same is true for albumin infusions.

Loop diuretics and aldosterone antagonists sometimes initiate a diuresis and should be tried.

🔵 Hepatopulmonary syndrome is a complication of cirrhosis caused by arteriovenous anastomoses in the lung, resulting in dyspnea and hypoxemia.

Pulmonary vascular vasodilation appears to be the cause. The A-V malformations can be diagnosed by bubble studies that demonstrate a right to left shunt. There is no effective treatment.

CARCINOID TUMORS

Carcinoid Tumors and the Malignant Carcinoid Syndrome

Carcinoid tumors are most commonly derived from enterochromaffin cells in the gut (Table 11-4). The enterochromaffin cells, in turn, are part of a larger group of diffuse neuroendocrine cells that are widely distributed in tissues derived from the embryologic foregut, midgut, and hindgut as well as in various endocrine glands. These cells have the unique capacity to take up biogenic amine precursors, decarboxylate them to the corresponding biogenic amine, and store the amine in granules within the cell along with peptides and polypeptides, some of which are recognized as classic hormones, as well as a variety of other enzymes and mediators. They have been referred to as APUD cells based on these histochemical features (Amine Precursor Uptake and Decarboxylation). Serotonin (5-hydroxytryptamine [5HT]) is the major biogenic amine produced by carcinoid tumors. Release of 5HT and peptide components of these cells give rise to the carcinoid syndrome.

🔵 Carcinoid tumors are among the most common neoplasms of the small bowel. The appendix and the ileum are the most common sites of origin. They incite a dense desmoplastic reaction that involves the mesentery and may be the cause of intestinal obstruction. Carcinoid tumors metastasize principally to the liver, but also to bone.

TABLE 11.4 The Classic Malignant Carcinoid Syndrome

Hepatomegaly

Extensive metastases

Flushing

Kallikrein (serine protease) from the tumor cleaves kininogens → vasodilatory peptides (like bradykinin); stimulated by β-adrenergic agonists

Diarrhea

Serotonin (5HT)

Hypotension

Bradykinin and other vasodilatory peptides; accentuated by catecholamines

Telangiectasias

Chronic vasodilatation

Right-sided cardiac lesions

Pulmonic stenosis and tricuspid regurgitation; 5HT and kinins

Wheezing

5HT, kinins, prostaglandins from the tumor

Pellagra

Tryptophan diversion → pellagra (dermatitis, dementia, diarrhea)

Diagnosis

↑ 24 hour urinary 5HIAA excretion

The small bowel is the most common site of carcinoid tumors; these originate from the embryologic midgut and account for about two-thirds of carcinoid tumors. Carcinoids also occur in structures derived from the foregut (thorax, stomach, about 25%) and hindgut (colon, rectum).

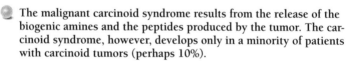

The malignant carcinoid syndrome results from the release of the biogenic amines and the peptides produced by the tumor. The carcinoid syndrome, however, develops only in a minority of patients with carcinoid tumors (perhaps 10%).

Appendiceal carcinoids are associated with appendicitis but not with the carcinoid syndrome.

The carcinoid syndrome is diagnosed by measuring the 24-hour excretion of 5-hydroxyindole acetic acid (5-HIAA), the major metabolite of serotonin.

Small intestinal carcinoids, principally arising in the ileum, produce the classic malignant carcinoid syndrome; carcinoids arising in the lungs or the stomach produce atypical or variant carcinoid syndromes. Carcinoids originating in the lung (bronchial carcinoids) may be deficient in the decarboxylase that forms 5-HIAA from 5-hydroxytryptophan (5-HTP) necessitating the measurement of 5-HTP in these cases.

 Carcinoids arising in the small intestines cause the carcinoid syndrome only after hepatic metastases have been established, since the liver metabolizes the released biologically active compounds; after metastases the tumor products gain access to the systemic circulation via the hepatic vein and produce the pathologic changes seen in the carcinoid syndrome.

 The major manifestations of the classic malignant carcinoid syndrome include hepatomegaly, flushing, diarrhea, wheezing, telangiectasias, hypotension, and cardiac valvular lesions.

The hepatomegaly reflects extensive metastatic infiltration of the liver. The diarrhea is a consequence of serotonin which increases intestinal contraction, shortens transit time, and produces abdominal cramping and, sometimes, malabsorption.

The characteristic flush lasts a few minutes and occurs in the typical blush areas; face, neck, and upper torso. It is reddish or purple in color and associated with a fall in blood pressure. It is a *faux pearl* that the carcinoid syndrome is a cause of secondary hypertension.

 The flush is not caused by 5HT; it is the result of kallikrein release from the tumor. Kallikrein is a serine protease that produces bradykinin and other vasodilatory peptides from their protein precursors in plasma.

The vasodilation causes the flush and the hypotension.

 Flushing in the malignant carcinoid syndrome may occur spontaneously or be induced by foods, alcohol, or catecholamines which release kallikrein from the tumor by a beta-adrenergic mechanism.

This may cause a big problem when surgery is performed on patients with the carcinoid syndrome and catecholamines are administered for hypotension. A paradoxical fall in BP which may be prolonged and severe is often the result. Pretreatment and intraoperative administration of the somatostatin analog octreotide is very useful since somatostatin analogs effectively block the release of vasoactive compounds from the tumor.

Telangiectasias may be the consequence of prolonged vasodilation. Brawny edema may also occur involving the face and extremities.

Wheezing may reflect the release of bronchospastic-inducing compounds such as 5HT, prostaglandins, kinins, and prostaglandins. Treatment with beta-adrenergic agonists should be avoided as noted above.

Right-sided cardiac lesions occur in up to 50% of patients with the carcinoid syndrome over the course of the disease. Cardiac involvement consists of subendocardial fibrosis which results in tricuspid regurgitation and pulmonic stenosis.

The right-sided location of the lesions reflects the direct application of serotonin and perhaps bradykinin to the endocardium from the hepatic vein. Left-sided lesions are much less common since the bioactive compounds are inactivated during passage through the lungs.

The cardiac lesions of the carcinoid syndrome resemble those induced by the weight loss drug d-fenfluramine. The latter works by releasing serotonin from central neurons that regulate appetite, thus implicating serotonin in the pathogenesis of the cardiac lesions associated with the carcinoid syndrome.

 Tryptophan diversion in patients with a large tumor burden may result in niacin deficiency and manifestations of pellagra.

Normally, about 1% of dietary tryptophan goes to 5HT synthesis, but in patients with the malignant carcinoid syndrome up to 70% of tryptophan may be diverted to the serotonin pathway, resulting in diarrhea, hyperpigmented skin lesions, and mental status changes. Patients with advanced disease frequently have a masked facies and flat affect. Protein deficiency with hypoalbuminemia may develop as well.

 Carcinoid tumors originating from the embryologic foregut have variant manifestations that differ from the classic carcinoid syndrome.

Foregut carcinoids may occasionally produce the syndrome without hepatic metastases by drainage directly into the systemic circulation.

Gastric carcinoids have a red pruritic rash that may reflect the release of histamine from the tumor. Bronchial carcinoids that produce the syndrome are associated with intense flushing that may last hours to days in association with lacrimation and salivation.

 Bronchial carcinoids may secrete ACTH and constitute an important cause of the ectopic ACTH syndrome.

Small cell carcinoma of the lung is the highly malignant neuroendocrine variant of the bronchial carcinoid tumor.

Obesity *12*

PATHOGENESIS OF OBESITY

The striking increase in the prevalence of obesity over the last few decades, coupled with the greater appreciation of the major role that obesity plays in development of many acute and chronic diseases, has rekindled interest in the pathogenesis of the obese state. Is it strictly "gluttony and sloth," more calories and less activity, or do the obese differ in metabolic efficiency, rendering them prone to weight gain and its consequences?

 Obesity may be viewed as the direct consequence of traits evolved to avoid starvation.

These traits affect appetite and energy expenditure ensuring adequate intake during periods of abundance and diminished expenditure of energy during famine.

The Energy Balance Equation

Any consideration of obesity should begin with the simple tautologic expression known as the energy balance equation, given below.

Energy intake = Energy output + storage

Although superficially simple, each of the components of the equation is more complicated than it seems. Energy intake is food consumed but it is now recognized that gut bacteria, the microbiome, are involved in nutrient processing in ways that favor or antagonize weight gain. Compounds produced by the microbiome may also influence metabolism by pathways that are currently unrecognized. Both the micro- and the macronutrient content of the diet also play a role. Although energy intake is, thus, more than just calories ingested, appetite obviously plays a crucial role by regulating food intake.

 The regulation of appetite involves a complex series of signals from the periphery and within the CNS; these stimulatory and inhibitory factors interact at the level of the hypothalamus to regulate energy intake.

171

The orexigenic pathways in the arcuate nucleus of the hypothalamus involve the Agouti-related peptide (AgRP) and the neurotransmitter neuropeptide y (NPY) while the anorexigenic ones involve pro-opiomelanocortin (POMC) which includes melanocyte-stimulating hormone (MSH), the endogenous ligand for the melanocortin-4 receptor (MC4R) and serotonin (5HT). Leptin, the polypeptide product of the *ob/ob* gene, is secreted by adipocytes and suppresses appetite by inhibiting the orexigenic pathways and stimulating the anorexigenic ones.

The components of this system represent potential druggable targets for the treatment of obesity if the obstacle of off-target effects, particularly those in the CNS, can be overcome.

🔵 **Energy output, once equated with physical activity alone, is now recognized to include important inter-individual differences in basal metabolic rate (BMR) and in the efficiency with which ingested calories are utilized and stored.**

BMR accounts for between 60% and 80% of total energy output depending on the level of physical activity. BMR is the heat generated from tissue metabolism throughout the body. About 10% of daily energy expenditure represents "adaptive" thermogenesis, generated by SNS stimulation of brown adipose tissue (BAT).

🔵 **Fat storage depots, once considered inert energy repositories, are now recognized to produce a large variety of biologically active compounds that influence metabolism and the propensity for weight gain.**

Leptin is a good example: synthesized in adipose tissue and reflective of an individual's fat mass, leptin feeds back to the hypothalamus to suppress appetite and stimulate the sympathetic nervous system (SNS) which increases energy expenditure. Leptin, therefore, is involved in the maintenance of energy balance by affecting both the intake and the output sides of the energy balance equation.

🔵 **Overfeeding studies have demonstrated conclusively that individuals differ in metabolic efficiency (the relationship between ingested calories and storage of fat).**

When overfed a measured increase in caloric intake for significant periods of time individuals vary in the amount of weight gained. Some gain incrementally, close to the calculated caloric excess, while others dissipate more than half of the calories taken in excess. Overfeeding studies with pairs of twins show greater variation between twin pairs than within twin pairs, consistent with a genetic contribution to metabolic efficiency.

🔵 **Studies indicate that genetic factors contribute between 40% and 50% to the development of obesity.**

Thus, both the environment and genetics contribute to the pathogenesis of obesity.

Thrifty Metabolic Traits

Metabolic efficiency is one of several "thrifty" metabolic traits, evolved to resist death from starvation. These thrifty traits include lower metabolic rate, increased metabolic efficiency, and insulin resistance.

Lower BMR and more efficient metabolism resist death from starvation by decreasing the overall need for metabolizeable substrates. Insulin resistance diminishes the need for gluconeogenesis by diverting glucose from muscle which can utilize fat derived substrates, to the brain which requires glucose.

The cause of death in starvation is pneumonia, a consequence of muscle protein depletion which impairs the ability to cough and thus clear secretions from the upper airway.

The result is aspiration and death from pneumonia, as pointed out decades ago by Harvard Professor George Cahill.

In starvation gluconeogenesis is the only means of providing the brain with glucose, for practical purposes the only energy source the CNS is able to utilize.

Gluconeogenic precursors come from the breakdown of protein, of which skeletal muscle is the largest reservoir.

Insulin resistance, defined as a decrease in insulin-mediated glucose uptake in skeletal muscle, directs glucose away from muscle toward the brain, thus sparing muscle protein breakdown.

Thrifty metabolic traits, evolved to prolong survival during famine, promote the development of obesity and type 2 diabetes mellitus when the food supply is abundant.

Those individuals well supplied with thrifty traits would survive famine better but are heir to obesity and type 2 DM in developed countries today. These thrifty traits have persisted since the adverse effects of obesity develop over decades, well past reproductive age in most subjects. This is in distinction to starvation which has its effects in the short term.

Examples of the impact of thrifty traits on the development of obesity may be found in indigenous populations worldwide. The aboriginal people of Australia, the Maoris of New Zealand, and the Pima Indians of the southwest US, all of which faced bare subsistence conditions for centuries, were known to be thin 100 years ago, and now are plagued by obesity and its complications.

Successful treatments for obesity should address both sides of the energy balance equation: appetite and energy expenditure.

CARDIOVASCULAR AND METABOLIC CONSEQUENCES OF OBESITY

Most organ systems are adversely affected by obesity. In some, obesity plays a major role in disease risk; in others, a contributory factor. Obesity has a dominant role in the development of cardiovascular disease, both directly and as a consequence of its role in the causation of type 2 DM and hypertension.

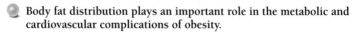 **Body fat distribution plays an important role in the metabolic and cardiovascular complications of obesity.**

Body mass index (BMI) and percent body fat are important indices of obesity but do not tell the whole story. The distribution of fat between upper body (central, abdominal) and lower body (gluteal) has been referred to as android (apple shaped) and gynoid (pear shaped) respectively, although the fat distribution is not specific for gender. Both men and women may have either type of distribution. Jan Vague, a French clinician practicing in the middle of the last century, coined the terms android and gynoid and noted that the metabolic (diabetes) and the cardiovascular complications of obesity (hypertension, myocardial infarction) tracked with the android form of obesity.

Using surrogate measures such as waist circumference or waist to hip ratio it has been firmly established that the upper body (android) form of obesity is associated with greater insulin resistance and hyperinsulinemia than the lower body form (gynoid). Insulin resistance, thus, tracks with the metabolic and cardiovascular complications of obesity. Fat within the abdomen, and in the liver seem to play and important role in the genesis of complications associated with obesity.

It is not clear what determines the distribution of body fat. Since intra-abdominal adipocytes are more sensitive to hormonal stimulation than adipocytes from peripheral sites, insulin-stimulated lipogenesis may be involved.

The activation of a glucocorticoid effect in intra-abdominal adipocytes by the action of 5-hydroxysteroid dehydrogenase is another possible mechanism; favoring the formation of active cortisol relative to inactive cortisone in abdominal adipocytes might be associated with expansion of the abdominal fat mass as seen in Cushing's syndrome.

Abdominal (central, android) obesity is the major cause of insulin resistance.

Although insulin has many actions in the regulation of metabolism insulin resistance refers specifically to its effect on skeletal muscle uptake of glucose, since more than 80% of total body glucose uptake mediated by insulin goes into skeletal muscle. The insulin resistance is caused by lipid accumulation in muscle which blocks the translocation of the glucose transporter (GLUT 4) to the cell membrane, a necessary prerequisite for transport of glucose into the cell.

Hyperinsulinemia is a consequence of insulin resistance.

The impediment to glucose uptake raises the blood glucose level stimulating more insulin release from the pancreatic beta cells and establishing a new steady state with a normal to slightly elevated glucose level and an elevated level of insulin. When the beta cells can no longer keep up with the demand imposed by insulin resistance plasma glucose rises and impaired glucose tolerance followed by type 2 DM ensues.

Another theory postulates that hyperinsulinemia is primary, since it has been known for a long time that elevated insulin levels induce insulin resistance.

- **Many of the adverse effects of obesity are rooted in insulin resistance.**

- **Obesity, particularly the abdominal form, is the major risk factor for the development of both type 2 DM and hypertension.**

Insulin resistance with pancreatic failure leads to type 2 DM. Hypertension results from SNS stimulation driven by hyperinsulinemia and leptin, coupled with a direct effect of insulin on the renal tubular reabsorption of sodium.

- **High triglycerides and low HDL cholesterol constitute the characteristic dyslipidemia of obesity.**

Population-based studies demonstrate that insulin plays a major role in the genesis of the obesity-related dyslipidemia.

- **Acanthosis nigricans is a dermatologic marker of hyperinsulinemia.**

A velvety, verrucous pigmented lesion located behind the neck, in the axillae, and on the knuckles may occur in insulin-resistant states, perhaps because hyperinsulinemia stimulates epidermal growth factor receptors.

- **Insulin resistance, abdominal obesity, hypertension, and high triglycerides – low HDL, form a cluster known as "the metabolic syndrome."**

A better name for this constellation would have been the "insulin resistance syndrome" since insulin is the thread that ties these diverse manifestations together. The following may also be associated: small dense (atherogenic) LDL; microalbuminuria; type 2 DM; hyperuricemia; coagulation abnormalities (increased plasminogen activator inhibitor-1, PAI-1); nonalcoholic fatty liver disease (NAFLD); and increased inflammatory markers.

Although arguments abound as to whether this is a distinct syndrome, the clinical significance of this cluster is the enhanced cardiovascular risk that the various components confer.

- **The obesity paradox: longevity, including longevity in a variety of chronic disease, is greater in the overweight (BMI 25 to 30) and the modestly obese (BMI 30 to 33). There is a "J" curve relationship between obesity and mortality.**

The reasons for this counterintuitive finding are not entirely clear. In part it may be that obesity itself without the confounding effects of diabetes or hypertension has a mild protective effect. The presence of hypertension and/or diabetes, of course, has a detrimental effect on longevity.

Since this direct relationship between BMI and mortality is stronger in the elderly, what the epidemiologists refer to "survivor bias" or "depletion of susceptibles" (those at risk die earlier) may be involved.

OBESITY AND OTHER DISEASES

Obesity exerts adverse effects on virtually all organ systems. In addition to the cardiovascular system and impaired carbohydrate tolerance outlined above, the most important organ systems or diseases impacted by obesity include the liver, the joints, the gut, respiration, and malignancies.

> **NAFLD, "fatty liver," is increasingly recognized as an important complication of obesity since it may progress to NASH (nonalcoholic steatohepatitis) and thence to cirrhosis.**

Accumulation of fat in the liver is a critical component of the abdominal (central) obesity phenotype, and occurs frequently in patients with the metabolic syndrome. As such it is associated with, and predictive of, increased cardiovascular morbidity and mortality.

The increased levels of free fatty acids in obesity, coupled with hyperinsulinemia, leads to increased triglyceride synthesis in hepatocytes. In and of itself NAFLD is not serious and is rapidly reversible; the danger lies in the progression to NASH and cirrhosis.

> **NASH evolves when fat in the liver stimulates inflammatory cell infiltration.**

For reasons that are not entirely clear fat may trigger the release of proinflammatory cytokines from hepatocytes with resultant infiltration by inflammatory cells. The result is steatohepatitis which may be accompanied, in a minority of such patients, by fibrosis, loss of normal hepatic microarchitecture, and cirrhosis. The complications of cirrhosis that develops in patients with NASH are the same as those that complicate cirrhosis of other etiologies: portal hypertension, variceal hemorrhage, and hepatocellular carcinoma.

> **Osteoarthritis of the hips and knees, gastroesophageal reflux, sleep apnea, and polycystic ovarian syndrome complicate obesity.**

> **Certain malignancies are more common in the obese including all portions of the GI tract, pancreas, liver, gall bladder, breast, ovarian and endometrial carcinomas, prostate cancer, and lymphomas.**

The mechanisms are unclear but higher levels of insulin and insulin-like growth factors along with proinflammatory cytokines are potential factors.

Malignancy and Paraneoplastic Syndromes

13 CHAPTER

BRONCHOGENIC CARCINOMA

The three basic cell types of carcinoma of the lung – small cell (about 15%, of all lung cancers), adenocarcinoma (40%), and squamous cell (35%) – have distinct clinical features and are associated with different paraneoplastic syndromes. Large cell carcinoma of the lung (10% to 15%) is the term reserved for those carcinomas not meeting histologic criteria of the three classic types.

Although some tumors have a mixed histologic picture, particularly squamous and adenocarcinomas, distinct clinical features are the rule. The mixed tumors may reflect stem cell malignancy with differentiation into separate cell lines.

Lung Cancer Metastases

All bronchogenic carcinomas have the potential for widespread metastases, frequently involving bone and brain, and are associated with a poor prognosis.

Lung cancer shows a peculiar predilection for metastasis to the adrenals and pituitary.

Metastases to pituitary and adrenals are relatively common, but clinical manifestations are rare.

The posterior pituitary is the part of the gland most commonly involved, explaining the association of lung cancer with diabetes insipidus (DI); principally small cell carcinomas, but nonsmall cell carcinomas also cause this syndrome.

177

Carcinoma of the breast is the other tumor associated with DI. Adrenal metastases from lung cancer, although very common, only rarely cause adrenal insufficiency.

Smoking is, of course, the major risk factor for all types of lung cancer, but a significant minority of patients with adenocarcinoma have no smoking history. Asbestos exposure is also a risk factor for all types of lung cancer and the risk is compounded by smoking. Asbestos is the major cause of mesothelioma.

🔹 **Radiographically, lung cancer metastases to bone appear lytic but contain a small rim of osteoblastic activity and are therefore associated with an elevated alkaline phosphatase level (made by osteoblasts) and a positive bone scan.**

Superior Vena Cava (SVC) Syndrome

🔹 **Superior vena cava (SVC) syndrome, obstruction of blood flow in the SVC, is an important complication of both small and nonsmall cell lung cancer.**

Centrally located tumors, particularly those on the right side, are the usual cause. Lymphomas also may cause the SVC syndrome along with other diseases of the mediastinum including aneurysms, fibrosing disorders, and metastatic cancers.

The symptoms and signs are the predictable consequences of venous obstruction to the drainage of the head, neck, and upper thorax, including: plethora, facial edema and suffusion, increased venous pattern on the right chest, tortuous veins on funduscopic examination, and sometimes, papilledema in severe cases.

Digital Clubbing

🔹 **Digital clubbing occurs in over one-half of patients with nonsmall cell carcinoma of the lung.**

Clubbing, a spongy elevation of the base of the nail that obliterates the usual angle formed by the nail with its base, is associated, additionally, with a variety of different diseases including suppurative intrathoracic processes, cyanotic congenital heart disease, inflammatory bowel disease, and biliary cirrhosis among others.

🔹 **Clubbing is rare in small cell carcinoma of the lung and in uncomplicated TB.**

🔹 **The most exuberant clubbing occurs in patients with adenocarcinoma of the lung.**

Paraneoplastic Syndromes

Bronchogenic carcinomas are associated with a wide variety of paraneoplastic syndromes as noted in Table 13-1. Different cell types produce distinct syndromes with reasonable fidelity.

TABLE 13.1 Paraneoplastic Syndromes with Bronchogenic Carcinomas

Histologic Type	Paraneoplastic Syndrome
Adenocarcinoma	Hypertrophic pulmonary osteoarthropathy
	Trousseau's syndrome
Squamous cell carcinoma	Humoral hypercalcemia of malignancy (PTHrP)
	Pancoast syndrome
Small (oat) cell carcinoma	SIADH
	Lambert–Eaton myasthenic syndrome
	Cerebellar degeneration

Adenocarcinoma of the Lung

Adenocarcinomas of the lung tend to be peripheral in location (in contrast to the other types which tend to be central).

Bronchoalveolar carcinoma of the lung, a subtype of adenocarcinoma now referred to as carcinoma in situ because it does not invade the lung interstitium, is characterized by aerogenous spread via the bronchi; although the prognosis may be better than other types when localized, it may be associated with widespread disease throughout the lung fields, and a correspondingly poor prognosis.

Adenocarcinomas may develop in relation to parenchymal scars within the lungs – the so called "scar carcinoma."

These may occur in the area of old tuberculous scars.

Hypertrophic pulmonary osteoarthropathy, the subperiosteal deposition of new bone, occurs in association with exuberant clubbing, and is most common in association with adenocarcinoma of the lung.

A common clinical presentation is ankle pain and swelling although the wrists may occasionally be involved as well. Bone scan is diagnostic, showing subperiosteal enhancement in the long bones of the extremities.

It may be associated with a velvety thickening and pigmentation over the skin of the palms. The pathogenesis is not well understood but growth factors produced by the tumor are suspected to contribute.

Trousseau's syndrome, migratory superficial thrombophlebitis, is associated with adenocarcinoma of the lung.

Described by Armand Trousseau in the mid-19th century, and now recognized to be a manifestation of malignancy associated hypercoagulable state, thrombophlebitis may complicate adenocarcinoma of the lung. As a paraneoplastic syndrome the thrombophlebitis may antedate the clinical presentation of the tumor. Mucinous adenocarcinomas of the lung, the stomach, or the pancreas are the usual causes of this syndrome. Ironically, a few years after describing this entity Trousseau diagnosed it in himself and subsequently went on to die from pancreatic (some say gastric) carcinoma.

Arterial thromboses have been noted as well although some of those described may have been paradoxical emboli through a patent foramen ovale.

Squamous Cell Carcinoma of the Lung

● Originating centrally more commonly than in the periphery, squamous cell lung cancers frequently cavitate and may cause confusion with lung abscess.

As compared with lung abscesses the walls of a cavitated squamous carcinoma appear thicker and have a shaggy appearance.

● In an edentulous patient a cavitary lesion on chest x-ray is a carcinoma until proved otherwise.

Lung abscesses usually occur in conjunction with poor oral hygiene and periods of diminished consciousness.

● Squamous carcinomas originating in the apex of the lung (the "superior sulcus" or Pancoast tumor) are associated with a characteristic constellation of symptoms and signs known as Pancoast's syndrome.

The clinical manifestations result from local invasion of surrounding tissues including the brachial plexus, the superior cervical (sympathetic) ganglion, ribs and vertebral bodies.

● Gnawing pain in the neck, shoulder, and upper back, worse at night, may become unbearable; weakness and atrophy of the intrinsic muscles of the hand and Horner's syndrome reflect invasion of the ipsilateral nerve roots and the sympathetic paravertebral chain.

Disruption of the cervical components of the SNS causes miosis, ptosis, and anhydrosis – Horner's syndrome.

● Squamous cell cancer of the lung may be associated with a paraneoplastic syndrome known as humoral hypercalcemia of malignancy (HHM), caused by production and secretion of parathyroid hormone-related protein (PTHrP) by the tumor.

Hypercalcemia in association with malignancy has several causes: bony dissolution secondary to extensive osteolytic metastatic disease; cytokine activation of osteoclast activity; the production of calcitriol; and the production of PTHrP which results in the HHM syndrome. PTHrP, a homolog of parathyroid hormone (PTH) that reproduces some of the biologic actions of PTH, is the most common cause of hypercalcemia in solid tumors (absent known bone metastases) and is the usual cause of hypercalcemia in patients with squamous cell carcinomas.

Small Cell Carcinoma of the Lung

A highly aggressive malignancy derived from pulmonary neuroendo-crine cells, small cell carcinoma of the lung is usually widespread at the time of initial diagnosis.

Small cell carcinoma of the lung, previously known as oat cell carcinoma, is the malignant counterpart of the differentiated carcinoid tumor. It is extremely rare in those who have never smoked. Typically forming large central masses, small cell lung cancer is a common cause of SVC syndrome.

A number of distinct paraneoplastic syndromes are associated with small cell carcinoma of the lung, reflecting, perhaps, the neuroendo-crine origin of this tumor.

Syndrome of inappropriate ADH secretion (SIADH), ectopic ACTH syndrome, Lambert–Eaton syndrome, and cerebellar degeneration are all well recognized entities complicating small cell lung cancer. Treatments that destroy the tumor reverse the paraneoplastic syndromes.

SIADH may be caused by any intrathoracic process that stimulates, inappropriately, the release of ADH from the posterior pituitary. Some tumors, however, produce and secrete ADH directly, as is the case with small cell carcinoma of the lung.

In the presence of hyponatremia and low serum osmolality, a urine osmolality greater than plasma or less than maximally dilute is diagnostic of SIADH. The urinary sodium is generally high reflecting dietary intake.

The ectopic ACTH syndrome secondary to small cell carcinoma of the lung differs from other causes of Cushing's syndrome in several ways: weight loss rather than weight gain modifies the usual physical stigmata that depend on fat accumulation such as moon facies and buffalo hump; hypokalemic alkalosis, rare in other forms of Cushing's syndrome, dominates the clinical course; and hyper-pigmentation, due to very high ACTH levels, is usually present. Diabetes, hypertension, and muscle weakness are also prominent features.

The ACTH levels in the ectopic ACTH syndrome associated with small cell carcinomas of the lung are very high resulting in the production of a variety of mineralocorticoids (such as deoxycorticosterone) which cause the hyperten-sion and the hypokalemic alkalosis. Aldosterone is not increased.

The Lambert–Eaton myasthenic syndrome (LEMS) superficially resembles myasthenia gravis (MG) but is distinct on both clinical and pathophysiologic grounds. In the majority of cases LEMS is a paraneoplastic syndrome most commonly associated with small cell carcinoma of the lung; it also can occur without detectable cancer although vigilance is required since LEMS may antedate the appear-ance of cancer by years.

MG is an autoimmune disease caused by antibodies directed at the skeletal muscle cholinergic receptor; as a consequence the receptor is degraded and the muscle response diminishes with repeated nerve stimulation. LEMS is also associated with an autoantibody but with a different target: the voltage-gated calcium channel on the prejunctional neuronal membrane. This antibody blocks the calcium channel and antagonizes the release of acetylcholine from the presynaptic neuron.

> **The clinical features of LEMS in comparison with MG include greater lower extremity involvement, less ocular and bulbar involvement, enhanced muscle contraction with repeated stimulation rather than fatigue of the response.**

Antibodies to the voltage-gated calcium channel can be demonstrated in most patients with LEMS and are useful diagnostically similar to the percentage of patients with generalized MG that have cholinergic receptor autoantibodies; by contrast, only about 50% of patients with ocular MG have demonstrable antibodies to the cholinergic receptor.

> **Paraneoplastic cerebellar degeneration occurs most commonly with small cell carcinoma of the lung.**

The tumor is associated with autoantibodies directed against the Purkinje cells of the cerebellum. Lymphoma and breast cancer have also been associated with cerebellar degeneration.

> **Imaging studies are not helpful in diagnosing cerebellar degeneration except for ruling out other diseases affecting the cerebellum.**

> **The clinical features of paraneoplastic cerebellar degeneration are typical of those found in cerebellar dysfunction of other causes: nausea, vomiting, dizziness, ataxia, inability to walk or stand, and diplopia among others.**

The Lambert–Eaton syndrome and other forms of paraneoplastic degeneration may sometimes accompany the cerebellar degeneration.

RENAL CELL CARCINOMA

> **Renal cell carcinoma (hypernephroma) is commonly associated with systemic manifestations, some of which reflect the biologic effects of cytokines released from the tumor, others as manifestations of classic paraneoplastic syndromes.**

At the present time only a small minority of patients demonstrate the classic triad of hematuria, flank pain, and an abdominal mass at presentation. Systemic symptoms often dominate the clinical picture and the diagnosis is frequently made by imaging techniques which demonstrate a renal mass.

> **Fever, night sweats, and cachexia are common manifestations of renal cell carcinoma that reflect cytokine release. Anemia and thrombocytosis are common as well secondary to the chronic inflammatory state.**

Local spread into the vena cava and adjacent lymph nodes, and metastases to lung, bone, liver, and brain are common complications. The inflammatory state may also result in secondary (AA) amyloidosis.

- **The paraneoplastic complications of renal cell carcinoma include hypercalcemia, erythrocytosis, and hypertension.**

- **Hypercalcemia reflects both bony metastases and the secretion of PTHrP by the tumor.**

The metastases appear lytic on bone films but, like lung tumor metastases, an osteoblastic rim elevates the alkaline phosphatase and results in a positive radionuclide bone scan.

- **Erythropoietin production by the tumor is relatively common but erythrocytosis is only noted in a small minority of patients, a consequence, perhaps, of cytokine suppression of erythropoiesis.**

- **Hypertension also complicates renal cell carcinoma, likely a consequence of renin production by tumor cells or by compressed adjacent kidney parenchyma.**

MULTIPLE MYELOMA

- **Myeloma, a plasma cell malignancy, classically presents with bone pain and anemia. Lytic lesions in bone, a normal alkaline phosphatase, and an "M" spike on serum protein electrophoresis is virtually diagnostic of multiple myeloma, but the diagnosis is usually confirmed by bone marrow aspirate showing an excess of (immature) plasma cells and by measurement and quantification of immunoglobulin levels.**

Clonal expansion of plasma cells in the bone marrow, paraprotein spike in excess of 3 g, and increases in circulating and urinary light chains make the diagnosis.

- **The bone lesions in myeloma are purely lytic, so alkaline phosphatase is not elevated and bone scans are unrevealing.**

The lytic lesions are caused by the production of osteoclast-activating factors, a variety of cytokines that stimulate osteoclasts and inhibit osteoblasts.

Pathologic fractures are an important complication of myeloma; they may involve vertebrae and/or long bones.

- **Persistent low back pain, often mistaken for degenerative lumbosacral spine disease, is a frequent presentation, especially in the elderly.**

The coincidental finding of anemia (normochromic, normocytic) in a patient with unrelenting low back pain indicates the need for further workup.

The lumbar spine is most commonly involved in compression fractures due to myeloma, although any area of the spine may be affected. Osteoporotic fractures, in contrast, most commonly involve the thoracic spine.

Hypercalcemia occurs in a significant proportion of cases due to bony dissolution in conjunction with immobilization due to pain.

Glucocorticoids are an important component of the treatment of the hypercalcemia.

Renal Involvement in Myeloma

Renal insufficiency in myeloma is common and involves several distinct pathogenetic mechanisms: light chain cast nephropathy ("myeloma kidney") is the most common.

Myeloma kidney is due to intratubular obstruction by filtered light chains that precipitate in the renal tubules and damage the tubular epithelium.

Bence Jones proteinuria, now of historical interest, was a test for myeloma that depended on the precipitation of the urinary light chains when the urine was heated followed by solubilization of the protein precipitate as the heating was continued. Direct determination of clonal light chains in plasma and urine has replaced the test for Bence Jones proteins.

Radiologic contrast media may precipitate light chains in the urine and result in acute renal failure; x-ray contrast media should be avoided in all patients with suspected myeloma.

Nonsteroidal anti-inflammatory drugs (NSAIDs) should be avoided as well.

Additional causes of azotemia in patients with myeloma include amyloidosis (AL), hypercalcemia, and mesangial deposition of light chains.

Severe renal involvement is a poor prognostic sign in patients with myeloma.

Impaired Antibody Production in Myeloma

All patients with myeloma have deficient antibody production, an acquired form of hypogammaglobulinemia despite elevated globulin levels. As such they are subject to severe and sometimes recurrent infections, most often with encapsulated organisms.

Since antibody-mediated opsonization is critical to host defenses against encapsulated organisms all patients with functional hypogammaglobulinemia are at risk for infections with pneumococci and *Klebsiella,* staphylococci, and *Escherichia coli.* The usual sites of infection are the lungs (pneumonia) and the kidneys (pyelonephritis).

Patients with chronic lymphocytic leukemia (CLL) are at similar risk since they are functionally hypogammaglobulinemic as well.

TABLE 13.2 Plasma Cell Dyscrasias and Related Paraproteins

Disease Entity	Paraprotein (All Clonal)
Multiple myeloma	Immunoglobulin "M" spike + light chains
Plasmacytoma	"M" spike in about 50%
Monoclonal gammapathy of uncertain significance (MGUS)	"M" spike of less than 3 g/dL
Primary amyloidosis (AL)	Light chains
Waldenstrom's macroglobulinemia	IgM "M" spike
POEMS syndrome (osteoblastic myeloma)	"M" spike with lambda light chains
Heavy chain disease	Immunoglobulin heavy chain moiety

Plasma Cell Dyscrasias Related to Myeloma

🔵 Other plasma cell dyscrasias include solitary plasmacytomas and monoclonal gammopathies of uncertain significance (MGUS) (Table 13-2).

Plasmacytomas are malignant plasma cell tumors, usually solitary, that occur in the skeleton or soft tissues. Bone marrow and skeleton are otherwise normal and paraprotein is usually absent or present in low concentration. They are usually responsive to radiation therapy. An "M" spike (paraprotein) is present in about 50% of cases.

MGUS refers to patients with a monoclonal spike of less than 3 g/dL, no bone lesions, and no increase in plasma cells in the bone marrow. Patients with MGUS need to be followed because a small percentage will develop myeloma (1% to 2% per year).

Patients with "M" spikes greater than 3 g/dL and increased marrow plasma cells but no bone lesions, no anemia, normal calcium, and normal renal function, are sometimes considered to have "smoldering myeloma."

🔵 Diseases related to, but distinct from myeloma, include Waldenstrom's macroglobulinemia, Polyneuropathy, Organomegaly, Endocrinopathy, M protein, Skin changes (POEMS) syndrome (osteoblastic myeloma), and heavy chain disease.

Waldenstrom's Macroglobulinemia

🔵 Classified as a lymphoplasmacytic lymphoma that originates from B-lymphocytes in the bone marrow, Waldenstrom's macroglobulinemia is associated with an IgM paraprotein that increases the serum viscosity.

The sedimentation rate is very high because rouleaux formation is exuberant in the face of the IgM paraprotein.

> **The symptoms of hyperviscosity include headache, confusion, mucosal bleeding, hypoxia from sludging of blood, tissue ischemia, and interference with platelet function.**

Waldenstrom's macroglobulinemia accounts for most cases of hyperviscosity; plasmapheresis is the usual treatment. The disease is indolent with a favorable prognosis.

Hepatosplenomegaly may occur along with peripheral neuropathy but bone disease and renal disease are absent.

> **POEMS syndrome is an obscure constellation of findings linked to myeloma by the presence of a paraprotein and osteosclerotic bone lesions.**

Sensorimotor neuropathy with high CNS protein, and frequently papilledema, hepatosplenomegaly, impotence, gynecomastia, or amenorrhea, "M" spike with clonal lambda light chains, and hyperpigmentation, hyperhidrosis, and clubbing are the major manifestations.

Also known as the Crow–Fukase, or Takatsuki syndrome, most (but not all) of the reported cases have been from Japan or in patients of Japanese descent. The pathogenesis is unknown but the M paraprotein, various cytokines, and growth factors have been postulated to play a role.

Heavy Chain Disease

> **Heavy chain disease refers to a group of very rare plasmalymphocytic malignancies characterized by production of paraproteins that consist solely of the heavy chain moiety of immunoglobulins.**

The isolated heavy chains of IgA, IgG, and IgM constitute the paraprotein which serves as a marker for three distinct plasmalymphocytic malignances associated with different clinical manifestations.

This group is distinct from Waldenstrom's macroglobulinemia described above.

The IgA subtype is a form of GI mucosa-associated lymphoid tissue (MALT) lymphoma. The IgG subtype, known as Franklin's disease, is a lymphoproliferative disease with systemic symptoms and palatal and uvula edema from involvement of Waldemeyer's ring of pharyngeal lymphoid tissue. The IgM subtype resembles CLL.

Neuromuscular Disease 14 CHAPTER

HEADACHE

Headaches are common in young folks but not in the elderly. A new headache in mid to old age should always be taken seriously. In the elderly a new headache should raise the suspicion of temporal (also known as cranial) arteritis, and prompt evaluation with a sedimentation rate (ESR), which is typically very high.

Temporal (Cranial) Arteritis

Temporal arteritis is a granulomatous giant cell arteritis (GCA) involving the extracranial branches of the aorta that is associated with headache, fever, and a very high sedimentation rate.

Jaw claudication during mastication (masseter muscle ischemia) is a specific symptom that is very useful diagnostically.

The feared complication of temporal arteritis is blindness from involvement of the ophthalmic circulation.

Visual symptoms with headache should be considered a medical emergency. Temporal artery biopsy frequently (but not always) secures the diagnosis of GCA. High-dose steroid (60-mg prednisone per day) is effective treatment. The dose is tapered down following symptoms and ESR. Remission usually occurs after 1 or 2 years.

Migraine

Migraine is a vascular headache (vasoconstriction, followed by vaso-dilation) that usually begins at an early age. The pain results from the stretching of receptors in the adventitia of extra- and intracranial vasculature. Migraine is unilateral (favoring predominantly one side) and throbbing.

Nausea and vomiting are frequent; visual aura may be present (scintillating scotomata).

Migraine is worsened by alcohol ingestion, pregnancy, and oral contraceptive use. Some foods may trigger attacks.

Untreated, prolonged attacks may not be relieved until awakening after sleep. Neurologic signs and symptoms may occur (hemiplegic migraine), with or without the headache, reflecting the vasoconstriction.

Migraine frequently occurs after a stressful period is resolved (the Friday afternoon headache) in distinction to tension headache which occurs during the stress.

Migraine may be more common in left-handed people although this is controversial. It may also be associated with an autoimmune diathesis. Migraineous attacks may be preceded by a period of hypomania.

Tension Headache

Tension headaches are associated with muscle spasm in the neck and scalp.

The pain is felt as a constricting band in association with neck stiffness. In contrast to migraine alcohol ingestion tends to relieve the pain. Tension headaches may trigger migraines and *vice versa*.

Headaches with Increased Intracranial Pressure

Headaches caused by brain tumors (increased intracranial pressure [ICP]) usually do not interfere with sleep but are typically present on awakening.

Any headache present on awakening should raise suspicion of increased ICP.

The so-called hypertensive headaches are occipital in location and also present on awakening. These may reflect nocturnal increases in ICP and usually signify severe or malignant hypertension.

Most headaches noted in hypertensive patients reflect the unrelated simultaneous occurrence of two common diseases.

The presence of venous pulsations in the eye grounds categorically rules out increased ICP; the absence of these is not evidence of increased pressure unless it was known for certain that these had been present previously.

Venous pulsations are yet another demonstration of the importance of establishing a baseline of physical findings.

Headache secondary to sinus congestion has a peculiar predilection for the mid to late afternoon for reasons that remain obscure.

Nasal decongestants relieve this type of headache.

Headache is the predominant symptom of idiopathic intracranial hypertension (pseudotumor cerebri).

This disorder of young women, frequently associated with obesity, also causes diplopia, visual symptoms, and if severe threatens sight from pressure on the optic nerves. Imaging reveals slit-like ventricles and frequently an "empty" sella.

The syndrome is caused by defective clearance of CSF and acetazolamide is effective treatment in many cases.

Normal Pressure Hydrocephalus (NPH)

Although not typically associated with headache, NPH, like pseudotumor cerebri, is a disorder of CSF clearance, presumably at the level of the arachnoid granulations. As a consequence the ventricles enlarge impinging on the cortex and subcortical structures.

The classic triad of NPH is gait disturbance, incontinence, and dementia.

Diagnosis depends on imaging and the response to CSF drainage.

CT and MRI of the brain in NPH show dilated ventricles, no obstruction at the level of the aqueduct, and no enlargement of the sulci, the latter a distinguishing point between NPH and diffuse cortical atrophy.

Lumbar puncture with the removal of 30 to 50 mL of CSF often results in immediate, or sometimes delayed, improvement in gait and cognition. A ventricular peritoneal shunt provides long-term improvement in about 60% of patients.

NPH is important to recognize because it is a potentially reversible form of dementia.

ACUTE CEREBROVASCULAR EVENTS (STROKES)

Hypertension is the major risk factor for all cerebrovascular events.

The overwhelming majority of strokes (about 85%) are ischemic, the remainder being hemorrhagic. Noncontrast CT scan is the first study required in stroke patients to rule out intracerebral hemorrhage.

TABLE 14.1 Ischemic Strokes Involving the Cortex

Thrombotic	Embolic
Atherosclerosis (large vessels)	Atrial fibrillation
Occurs at night (awakens with deficit)	Occurs during the day
Stuttering onset; deficit evolves	Deficit maximal at onset
Obtundation (develops with large lesions)	Headache

Ischemic Strokes

🔹 Ischemic strokes are embolic or thrombotic; the territory served by the middle cerebral artery is most commonly affected.

The clinical features may often distinguish embolic and thrombotic strokes affecting the cerebral cortex (Table 14-1). Thrombotic strokes may be further subdivided into cortical and subcortical (white matter or lacunar infarcts).

🔹 Embolic strokes are of sudden onset, occur during the day, are frequently associated with headache, occasionally with a seizure, and the associated neurologic deficit is maximal at onset.

Emboli most frequently originate in the heart with atrial fibrillation as the major associated abnormality. Vegetations on the heart valves, recent myocardial infarction, or prosthetic heart valves are also important causes.

🔹 Paradoxical emboli result from venous thrombosis with embolization of clot through a patent foramen ovale.

Ultrasonic demonstration of both the venous thrombosis and a patent foramen ovale by cardiac echo with a bubble study establishes the diagnosis.

🔹 The sudden onset of Wernicke's (fluent) aphasia is virtually always embolic.

Speech in Wernicke's aphasia, although fluent in distinction to the halting speech of Broca's aphasia, is incomprehensible gibberish ("word salad").

🔹 Thrombotic stroke typically occurs at night during sleep; the patient wakes up with the deficit.

The deficit from a thrombotic stroke may evolve over the course of 1 or 2 days. If the affected area is large, edema around the lesion may result in somnolence in the days following the stroke with subsequent improvement in consciousness as the swelling subsides.

🔹 Strokes affecting the nondominant hemisphere (right parietal lobe in right-handed people with left-sided cerebral dominance) are associated with striking neglect of the affected side.

This is often obvious from the position of the patient in the bed, who lies turned away from the affected (left) side. Having the patient draw a clock makes a nice demonstration of the neglect – all the numbers are on the right side. Astereognosis and sensory extinction on the affected side may also be demonstrable. Neglect is an important factor that hinders rehabilitation of nondominant hemisphere strokes.

> **Watershed strokes result from ischemia in the territory at the junction of the anterior and posterior circulations; they typically occur in patients with cardiovascular disease after an episode of hypotension with attendant poor perfusion of these vulnerable areas.**

Cardiac surgery is a common cause of watershed lesions. Involvement of the occipital cortex (between the anterior and posterior circulations) may result in cortical blindness. In the latter, pupillary reactions are preserved while vision is seriously impaired. About 50% of patients with cortical blindness are unaware of, or deny, their loss of sight.

> **Lacunar infarcts result from occlusion of smaller penetrating arteries in the region of the basal ganglia and the internal capsule. Lacunes account for about one-quarter of all ischemic strokes.**

The occlusion may reflect structural abnormalities of the small vessels or atheromatous occlusion at the origin of the penetrating vessels from the major branches of the middle cerebral arteries or the circle of Willis. Hypertension is presumed to be the usual underlying cause.

> **Isolated motor weakness of the upper or lower extremity or the face is the most common deficit produced by lacunes, but pure sensory strokes, ataxia, and dysarthria also occur.**

Lacunes may also be silent.

Cerebral Hemorrhage

Three lesions account for the majority of intracranial and intracerebral hemorrhage: "berry" or saccular aneursyms; microaneursyms of Charcot and Bouchard; and cerebral amyloid angiopathy (CAA).

> **Subarachnoid hemorrhage is associated with severe ("thunderclap") headache, nuchal rigidity, and, frequently, reduced level of consciousness.**

Noncontrast CT establishes the diagnosis in the great majority of cases.

> **Funduscopic examination in patients with subarachnoid hemorrhage commonly reveals blurred disc margins and retinal hemorrhages occur in about 25% of cases.**

> **Rupture of a "berry" aneurysm is the usual cause of subarachnoid hemorrhage. Polycystic kidney disease and coarctation of the aorta are predisposing diseases.**

Resulting from a defect in the muscular wall of the artery, berry aneursyms are most common in first or second order branches of arteries arising from the circle of Willis; the great majority are located in the anterior circulation.

 The microaneursyms of Charcot and Bouchard are important causes of intracerebral hemorrhage. These tiny aneurysms originate from very small arteries most commonly in the region of the basal ganglia (lenticulostriate arteries).

Antecedent hypertension is the usual cause. These microaneursyms are distinct from the larger berry aneurysms that cause subarachnoid hemorrhage.

Acute cerebellar hemorrhage is a medical emergency; prompt recognition followed by surgical evacuation of the hematoma is lifesaving (Table 14-2).

Like other intracerebral hemorrhages, the cause of cerebellar hemorrhage appears to be rupture of tiny microaneursyms as described by Charcot and Bouchard.

The clinical presentation of acute cerebellar hemorrhage includes the sudden onset of headache, vomiting, dizziness, and, particularly, the inability to stand or walk.

The inability to walk or even stand, with a tendency to fall backward is due to cerebellar ataxia and, along with intractable vomiting is an important clue to the diagnosis. Weakness of lateral gaze may be present as well. The disability usually progresses rapidly, so speed in diagnosis (noncontrast CT) and clot evacuation are critical. This is one instance where correct diagnosis and treatment results in cure without permanent disability but failure to diagnose and treat results in death. A high index of suspicion is necessary.

Cerebral amyloid angiopathy (CAA) is an important cause of intracerebral hemorrhage in the elderly. It is the usual cause in patients who have no history of hypertension.

TABLE 14.2 Acute Cerebellar Hemorrhage

Sudden onset
Headache
Vomiting
Dizziness
Inability to stand (truncal ataxia)
Unable to walk
Rapidly progressive downhill course

In comparison with the intracerebral hemorrhages associated with the micro-aneursyms of Charcot and Bouchard CAA hemorrhages are located more superficially in the cortex and subcortical areas rather than in the deeper brain structures. It may also occur in the cerebellum.

CAA is unrelated to systemic amyloidosis (AL, AA).

Drop Attacks

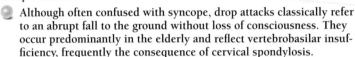 **Although often confused with syncope, drop attacks classically refer to an abrupt fall to the ground without loss of consciousness. They occur predominantly in the elderly and reflect vertebrobasilar insufficiency, frequently the consequence of cervical spondylosis.**

The vertebral arteries run through the transverse processes of the cervical vertebrae and are liable to kinking in the presence of cervical spine disease. Ischemia or compression of the brainstem or upper cord affects the posterior columns with transient loss of position sense and postural muscle tone. Evaluation should include imaging of the cervical spine. Elderly patients have trouble "finding their legs" and may have difficulty getting up after a drop attack.

WEAKNESS

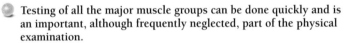 **Testing of all the major muscle groups can be done quickly and is an important, although frequently neglected, part of the physical examination.**

In addition to muscle testing careful assessment of the deep tendon reflexes and sensation is required. Hyperreflexia indicates an upper motor neuron or pyramidal (corticospinal) tract lesion. Flaccid paresis reflects lower motor neuron or primary muscle involvement.

Spinal Cord

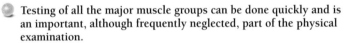 **Back pain and/or a sensory level, coupled with motor weakness and/or voiding difficulty imply spinal cord disease and necessitate immediate MRI of the spine.**

Encroachment of the spinal canal and compression of the cord by tumor or infection is a medical emergency that necessitates prompt imaging and treatment.

Myopathy

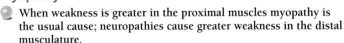 **When weakness is greater in the proximal muscles myopathy is the usual cause; neuropathies cause greater weakness in the distal musculature.**

Myopathies, excluding congenital dystrophies, are most commonly associated with endocrine or autoimmune diseases.

- Hyperthyroidism and Cushing's syndrome are common endocrine causes of proximal muscle weakness.

- Hypothyroidism causes stiffness rather than weakness and is frequently associated with high (sometimes very high) CPK levels.

- Weakness of the neck flexors is particularly prominent in dermato-myositis.

- Hypokalemic periodic paralysis, an autosomal dominant trait that is expressed more completely in men than in women, is frequently induced by large carbohydrate meals, or after a period of rest following strenuous exertion.

This inherited disorder of the voltage-gated calcium channel sometimes occurs in association with Graves' disease, especially in Asian men. Symptoms frequently occur in the morning after a period of intense exertion the previous day.

Guillain–Barre Syndrome

- Guillain–Barre syndrome (GBS), an immune-mediated polyradiculoneuropathy (usually following upper respiratory infection or campylobacter gastroenteritis), is an important cause of profound paralysis.

A variety of infections and occasionally vaccination have been associated with GBS. It typically begins in the lower extremities and spreads upward (Landry's ascending paralysis) and is often associated with autonomic instability (labile hypertension). The paralysis is flaccid and, except for parasthesias early in the course, does not affect sensation.

- The diagnosis is usually made clinically although it must be noted that many cases do not follow the typical ascending pattern and GBS should be considered in all cases of flaccid paralysis.

- Lumbar puncture gives the classic picture of "cytoalbuminemic dissociation" – high protein with slight, if any, pleocytosis.

EMG and nerve conduction studies may confirm the diagnosis, but, if nondiagnostic, treatment should not be delayed.

This disorder requires hospitalization for careful monitoring of the vital capacity since respiratory failure poses a significant threat. Early institution of plasmapheresis or IV gamma globulin is essential.

- The rare Miller Fisher variant of GBS consists of a triad of ophthalmoplegia, ataxia, and areflexia.

A different autoantibody with specificity for the third, fourth, and sixth cranial nerve appears to be involved.

Postviral Neurasthenia

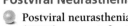 Postviral neurasthenia, also known as postviral fatigue syndrome (PVFS), or postinfectious fatigue syndrome (PIFS), is a poorly understood, but well-recognized syndrome characterized by overwhelming fatigue without demonstrable muscle weakness.

This chronic illness follows an infection, usually, but not exclusively, a viral infection, and usually, but not exclusively, upper respiratory in location. Sore throat is common in the predisposing illness. Infectious mononucleosis is the prototypic infection followed by a long period of fatigue but it is now recognized that PIFS may follow a variety of infections. Recovery from the acute episode is followed by physical and mental fatigue that interferes with the ordinary activities of daily living. PIFS is most common in young adults with a female predominance.

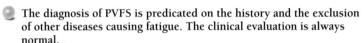 The diagnosis of PVFS is predicated on the history and the exclusion of other diseases causing fatigue. The clinical evaluation is always normal.

Although the symptoms suggest adrenal insufficiency adrenal testing is normal in these patients. This condition persists for months or sometimes a year or longer, but most patients improve over time with rest and rehabilitation. There is an overlap with "chronic fatigue syndrome," but the latter probably represents a less distinct and broader category of disease.

The pathogenesis of PVFS is not understood. It is not due to persistence of the original initiating infection, but may be a consequence of the immunologic response to the inciting agent. Chronic fatigue syndrome was originally hypothesized to represent persistent EBV infection, a theory now thoroughly discredited.

Myasthenia Gravis

Myasthenia gravis (MG), an autoimmune attack on the cholinergic receptors innervating striated skeletal muscle, typically involves the eyes (ptosis and diplopia) early in the course. The subsequent development of generalized disease occurs in the majority of cases.

The hallmark of MG is fatigue on repeated muscle contraction.

The eyes are most prominently involved in most (but not all) cases, presumably because of the high density of cholinergic receptors on the extraocular muscles and the eyelids.

Cold inactivates acetyl cholinesterase and a cold pack to the eye is a convenient test and much safer than the old tensilon test; relief of ptosis is a positive test and consistent with a diagnosis of MG.

Antibodies to the cholinergic receptor are confirmatory but these need not be present especially in the limited ocular form of the disease. The diagnosis of MG is largely clinical but EMG demonstrating diminished response with repeated stimulation confirms the diagnosis.

🔹 Thymoma has a well-recognized association with MG and needs to be ruled out; this association is most common in young women.

🔹 Limited disease (ocular myasthenia) is more common in older men and in patients with associated autoimmune thyroid disease.

Pyridostigmine provides symptomatic relief but immunosuppression is frequently required to control the disease and may prevent generalization after the onset with ptosis and diplopia alone.

🔹 Bulbar symptoms (impaired swallowing, phonation) are common as MG generalizes. These symptoms constitute a potential threat during upper respiratory infections since inability to clear secretions may cause respiratory failure.

Patients with MG presenting with an upper respiratory infection need a careful evaluation of bulbar function; the inability to clear oropharyngeal secretions poses a grave threat. Dysfunction of swallowing or phonation in conjunction with a respiratory infection necessitates in-hospital observation for impending respiratory failure.

🔹 A useful test of bulbar function is counting out loud up to 20 without taking a breath; inability to perform this or the development of a nasal twang as the counting progresses, indicates a dangerous depression of bulbar function and necessitates close observation in hospital.

Lambert–Eaton Myasthenic Syndrome (LEMS)

🔹 A paraneoplastic syndrome most commonly associated with small cell carcinoma of the lung, LEMS is associated with widespread muscle weakness that superficially resembles MG, but with important distinctive clinical features (Table 14-3).

In LEMS the antibody is directed at the voltage-gated calcium channel, and these antibodies may be demonstrated in about 50% of patients. Of particular note the muscle response to repetitive stimulation is enhanced in LEMS not diminished as it is in MG, and ocular and bulbar weakness is less prominent in LEMS as compared with MG.

Neuropathies

🔹 Polyneuropathy, formerly known by the synonymous term polyneuritis, is characterized by symmetrical dysfunction of sensory and motor nerves supplying the distal extremities. The causes are legion and include toxins, infections, metabolic abnormalities, vitamin deficiencies, drugs, and cancer, among others (Table 14-4).

TABLE 14.3 Myasthenic Syndromes

Myasthenia Gravis	Lambert–Eaton Syndrome
Autoantibody directed at nicotinic cholinergic receptors on skeletal muscle; blocks acetylcholine induced muscle contraction	Autoantibody directed at the voltage gated calcium channel on the prejunctional motor neuron; blocks the release of acetylcholine from the presynaptic neuron
Muscle response diminishes with repeated stimulation	Muscle response improves with repeated stimulation
Prominent ocular and bulbar involvement	Greater lower extremity involvement
Occasionally associated with thymoma (especially in young women)	Usually a paraneoplastic syndrome with small cell carcinoma of lung (may precede diagnosis of tumor)
Associated with autoimmune diathesis (thyroid, lupus, rheumatoid arthritis)	

Since the longest nerves are most vulnerable, the symptoms begin distally in the feet. Parasthesias, dysesthesias, and numbness are followed by flaccid weakness, areflexia, and, in severe cases, muscle atrophy. The distribution has been referred to as "stocking and glove" although the hands are not involved until the process has spread far up the legs. The diagnosis is clinical but may

TABLE 14.4 Peripheral Neuropathies

Polyneuropathy (Polyneuritis)	Mononeuritis Multiplex
Symmetrical dysfunction of distal somatic sensory and motor nerves	Infarction of one or more major motor nerves resulting in weakness of the muscles served
Parasthesias, dysesthesias, numbness, weakness	Cranial nerves often involved
Longer nerves most vulnerable (glove/stocking distribution)	Occlusion of the vasa nervorum by vasculitic, atherosclerotic, thrombotic, or infiltrative process is the proximate cause
Multiple causes including toxins, metabolic abnormalities, vitamin deficiencies, drugs, and malignancies	Underlying causes are limited and include diabetes, collagen vascular disease, malignancy

be confirmed by nerve conduction studies. High protein levels in the cerebro-spinal fluid are characteristic.

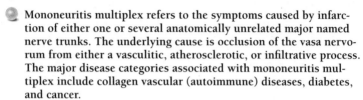 Mononeuritis multiplex refers to the symptoms caused by infarc-tion of either one or several anatomically unrelated major named nerve trunks. The underlying cause is occlusion of the vasa nervo-rum from either a vasculitic, atherosclerotic, or infiltrative process. The major disease categories associated with mononeuritis mul-tiplex include collagen vascular (autoimmune) diseases, diabetes, and cancer.

The usual presentation is the sudden onset of weakness in a major muscle nerve supplying a limb or cranial nerve. Sensation may be involved with pain in the nerve distribution but the hallmark is weakness. Spontaneous revas-cularization with recovery of function often occurs but takes a long time, frequently 1 or more years.

🔹 The collagen vascular diseases predisposing to mononeuritis multi-plex are, most commonly, polyarteritis nodosa, rheumatoid arthritis, Churg–Strauss syndrome, microscopic polyangiitis, and Wegener's granulomatosis.

Some infectious diseases such as Lyme disease and HIV may also be associated with mononeuritis multiplex.

Diabetic Neuropathy

🔹 In diabetics polyneuropathy is the most common form of peripheral nerve disease; when mononeuritis multiplex occurs in diabetics the cranial nerves of the extraocular muscles, most often the third cra-nial nerve, are frequent sites of involvement.

🔹 In long-standing diabetics the sudden onset of diplopia with the affected eye looking down (unopposed superior oblique) and out (unopposed lateral rectus) is a third nerve palsy rather than a stroke.

Ptosis is present as well. Pupillary reactions may not be affected since the nerves controlling the pupil are carried on the outside of cranial nerve III and therefore less subject to ischemia.

🔹 Diabetic amyotrophy is probably distinct from the other neuropa-thies and represents a painful lumbosacral plexopathy of unknown cause.

MOTOR NEURON DISEASE

Motor neuron disease refers to a neurodegenerative process of unknown cause that affects upper and lower motor neurons resulting in progressive paralysis.

Degeneration of lower motor neurons (anterior horn cells) and upper motor neurons (corticospinal neurons) gives rise to progressive weakness and muscle atrophy. The clinical features depend upon the pattern of nerve cell loss (upper vs. lower motor neurons) and the location of the muscles served by the degenerating neurons.

Weight loss and muscle atrophy are usually present at the time of presentation of motor neuron disease.

Amyotrophic Lateral Sclerosis (ALS)

The common form of the disease, ALS—Lou Gehrig's disease—results from degeneration in both anterior horn and corticospinal tract neurons.

Fasciculations and muscle atrophy reflect lower motor neuron degeneration; spasticity reflects upper motor neuron loss.

The diagnosis is clinical but may be confirmed by nerve conduction studies and EMG.

Fasciculations are the hallmark of motor neuron disease; they are caused by the depolarization of a dying anterior horn cell which causes contraction in the muscle fascicles served by that neuron (the motor unit).

As the degenerative process proceeds and more anterior horn cells die the fasciculations increase and spread to different parts of the body.

Not all fasciculations indicate motor neuron disease; benign calf fasciculations occur in normal people and are not a harbinger of motor neuron disease. Fasciculations in the upper extremities, particularly hands and shoulders, however, are almost always indicative of motor neuron disease.

Certain drugs, principally, depolarizing agents used in the induction of neuromuscular blockade, and cholinesterase inhibitors also cause fasciculations.

ALS is the prototype of motor neuron disease.

Anterior horn degeneration gives rise fasciculations and atrophy; corticospinal degeneration causes spasticity with hyperreflexia and positive Babinski sign. The disease is relentlessly progressive with death from respiratory failure. Interestingly cognition and ocular motility remain intact until the very end.

Differing patterns of motor neuron degeneration occur less commonly and involve principally the lower motor neurons (progressive or spinal muscular atrophy) or upper motor neurons (lateral column sclerosis).

The bulbar musculature may be involved as well with difficulty phonating and swallowing.

RHABDOMYOLYSIS

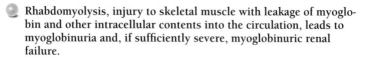 Rhabdomyolysis, injury to skeletal muscle with leakage of myoglo-bin and other intracellular contents into the circulation, leads to myoglobinuria and, if sufficiently severe, myoglobinuric renal failure.

Muscle damage from overexertion or external pressure is the usual cause although severe vasoconstriction with muscle ischemia can be associated as well.

Myoglobin in the urine produces a deep orange or brown color, useful in con-firming the diagnosis. Creatinine kinase (CK) levels are grossly elevated and may be in excess of 100,000 U/L.

Myoglobin causes acute renal failure by forming intratubular casts and damaging the renal tubular epithelium.

Other associated abnormalities include significant increases in serum phosphate, uric acid, and potassium. Hypocalcemia frequently occurs and may be prolonged.

Although originally described as part of the syndrome of crush injury, coma from drug overdose – with large areas of pressure necrosis – is now recognized as a significant cause of rhabdomyolysis and should be considered in patients found on the floor after suicide attempts or recreational drug use.

Bullous skin lesions around the areas of pressure in an unconscious patient found on the floor should suggest the possibility of rhabdo-myolysis.

The skin lesions are the consequence of pressure necrosis.

Cocaine use and pheochromocytoma with vasoconstrictive hyperten-sive crises have also been associated with rhabdomyolysis.

Severe muscle ischemia from catecholamine-induced vasoconstriction is an uncommon cause. The ischemia must be very severe and prolonged to cause muscle necrosis sufficient to produce rhabdomyolysis.

Neuroleptic malignant syndrome (NMS), characterized by hyperther-mia and extreme muscle stiffness in patients on neuroleptic agents, may be associated with rhabdomyolysis as well.

In patients with NMS the elevated temperature, as well as the intense muscle contraction, combine to produce rhabdomyolysis.

Alcohol excess, statin usage, and perhaps hypothyroidism may potentiate other causes of rhabdomyolysis or, less commonly, cause rhabdomyolysis on their own.

Diuresis with normal saline or, in the absence of contraindications, an alkaline diuresis should be initiated at the time of diagnosis. Dialysis may be necessary for high degrees of acute renal failure. Prognosis for recovery of renal function is good.

McArdle's Syndrome

McArdle's syndrome, an autosomal dominant inherited deficiency of muscle phosphorylase, is frequently associated with exertional muscle pain and rhabdomyolysis.

Also known as glycogen storage disease type V, the disease is characterized by muscle pain and stiffness on exertion due to inability to breakdown muscle glycogen. Although inherited it usually manifests in adult life after strenuous exertion. It is diagnosed by failure of exercising muscle to produce lactate since glycogenolysis is impaired. Genetic analysis may identify other cases within the family.

COMPLICATIONS OF PSYCHOTROPIC DRUGS

Parkinsonian features, eyes clenched tightly shut, lethargy, and confusion are highly suggestive of a reaction to neuroleptic agents.

Patients frequently present with a confusing array of symptoms, but the above features point strongly to drug effect.

Neuroleptic malignant syndrome (NMS) is a life-threatening reaction to the central dopaminergic blockade (D2 receptors) that occurs with a variety of psychotropic agents. It is characterized by mental status changes (confusion, delirium), high fevers, extreme muscle stiffness, and agitation.

The CPK is elevated, often to alarming levels, and rhabdomyolysis, as noted above, may occur with myoglobinuric renal failure. Supportive care in an ICU is required.

"Serotonin syndrome" is a severe reaction to serotonin excess at central nervous system synapses. Mental status changes, high fever, tachycardia, hypertension, and hyperreflexia are frequent findings.

Less muscle rigidity and the presence of prominent hyperreflexia often with lower extremity clonus, distinguish the serotonin syndrome from NMS. Drug withdrawal and supportive care are required.

In the elderly suspect drug effects when the clinical presentation is unusual and the list of prescribed medicines is long.

This is true for antiseizure medications and benzodiazepines as well as for neuroleptic agents. Dilantin overdose may be associated with a myriad of bizarre cerebellar signs. Measurement of drug levels and drug withdrawal clarify the situation.

Zoldipem (Ambien) is associated, in some patients, with bizarre behavior, sleepwalking, and other parasomnias.

Any of these behavioral manifestations preclude the subsequent use of Ambien.

SEIZURES

The etiology of a first grand malseizure differs according to the age at which it occurs.

- In young adults "idiopathic" epilepsy is the usual cause; in the sixth decade tumors, metastatic or primary CNS, are the most common etiology; in the seventh decade or later atherosclerotic disease (strokes and scars from strokes) is the predominant etiology.

- Elevation of the prolactin level (twice normal) 10 to 20 minutes after an attack supports the conclusion that a seizure has occurred.

Prolactin level returns to normal after 6 hours. Patients with vasovagal syncope may also have elevated prolactin levels but it is not clear whether this occurs only in those that have seizures with syncope (convulsive syncope). An elevated prolactin level is useful at distinguishing seizures from "pseudo seizures," a form of malingering.

Complications of Alcoholism

15 CHAPTER

Many of the complications of excessive alcohol intake (acute and chronic pancreatitis, alcoholic hepatitis and Laennec's cirrhosis, folate deficiency, scurvy, alcoholic ketoacidosis, and alcoholic hypoglycemia) have been dealt with in the appropriate organ system chapters.

NERVOUS SYSTEM

Chronic alcoholism exerts many adverse effects on both the peripheral and the central nervous system; some of these are due to direct toxic effects of ethanol; others reflect concomitant nutritional deficiencies that result from poor intake and/or gastrointestinal disease induced by alcohol. It is virtually impossible to distinguish the direct toxic effects from those caused by concomitant nutritional deficiency. Thiamine deficiency, in particular, is the nutritional factor related most closely to neurologic disorders associated with alcoholism.

Peripheral Nerves

 Chronic alcoholism is associated with a high incidence of peripheral sensorimotor neuropathy; sensory changes usually predominate.

Axonal degeneration, induced by alcohol or the alcohol metabolite acetaldehyde, or by nutritional deficiency, results in a typical symmetrical "glove and stocking" neuropathy that manifests with parasthesias, neuropathic pain, loss of deep tendon reflexes, and muscle weakness. Like all toxic and metabolic neuropathies nerve length determines the pattern of involvement: signs and symptoms begin in the feet and progress upward; the hands are not involved until the deficit in the lower extremities reaches the knee. Also, like the dysesthesias associated with other causes of neuropathy, pain is worse at night.

Central Nervous System

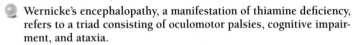 Wernicke's encephalopathy, a manifestation of thiamine deficiency, refers to a triad consisting of oculomotor palsies, cognitive impairment, and ataxia.

Thiamine (vitamin B_1) is an essential cofactor for the enzymes involved in carbohydrate metabolism. In the developed world thiamine deficiency affects principally chronic alcoholics although severe malnutrition from any cause may be associated with Wernicke's encephalopathy. In the early days of the AIDS epidemic, before effective treatment, thiamine deficiency was occasionally noted, with Wernicke's encephalopathy as the principal manifestation. The pathology includes petechial hemorrhages throughout the brainstem.

In vitamin-depleted alcoholics the administration of intravenous glucose may acutely precipitate Wernicke's encephalopathy by increasing the demand for thiamine when the supply is limited.

Glucose should never be administered to alcoholics without the concomitant administration of thiamine.

Bilateral sixth nerve palsy with failure of lateral gaze is the most common of the oculomotor manifestations and a defining characteristic of the syndrome although other oculomotor deficits may occur as well.

Both eyes crossed inwards results is a characteristic facial expression that reminds some observers of a Planaria worm. Nystagmus is frequently present but is not specific for Wernicke's encephalopathy.

The oculomotor palsies, if acute, may respond dramatically to intravenous thiamine with resolution immediately after the vitamin is administered. If the deficit has been present for a long time the response is less impressive or totally absent.

Ataxia in Wernicke's encephalopathy affects principally the gait and is due to a combination of peripheral neuropathy and degenerative changes in the vermis of the cerebellum.

Confusion, disorientation, and inattention are common signs of the mental changes in Wernicke's encephalopathy. The classic manifestation is the Korsakoff's syndrome.

Korsakoff's syndrome, also known as amnestic-confabulatory syndrome, is classically associated with Wernicke's, but may occur independently in chronic alcoholics.

The striking feature of Korsakoff's syndrome is amnesia for recent or current events with relative preservation of long-term memory. Classically, the patient with Korsakoff's syndrome fills in (confabulates) the amnestic deficits with made-up stories that can be elicited by the examiner (e.g., "how did you like the party last night?" which the patient responds to with elaborate made-up—confabulated—details).

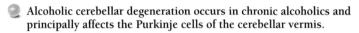 Alcoholic cerebellar degeneration occurs in chronic alcoholics and principally affects the Purkinje cells of the cerebellar vermis.

Lower extremity findings are more pronounced than upper extremity abnormalities and speech disorders although the latter may occur in severe cases.

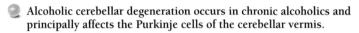 Alcohol-related dementia also occurs in association with diffuse cerebral atrophy.

The relationship to the Korsakoff's syndrome is uncertain but more generalized dementia occurs in some chronic alcoholics.

ALCOHOL WITHDRAWAL SYNDROMES

Alcohol is a potent CNS depressant. Adaptation to the depressed cerebral state results in a variety of excitatory changes when the depressive effect is abruptly removed by a decrease in alcohol intake. Sustained heavy drinking for a long time is necessary before pronounced withdrawal manifestations appear. Sympathoadrenal excitation is an important concomitant of severe alcohol withdrawal. There are three generally recognized and distinct withdrawal syndromes: seizures, alcoholic hallucinosis, and delirium tremens (DTs).

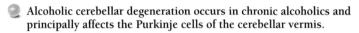 An alcohol withdrawal seizure usually occurs about 1 or 2 days after the last drink. The withdrawal seizure is typically generalized and single, although rarely, a brief burst of a few seizures may occur.

More than one seizure should raise the suspicion of a cause other than, or in addition to, alcohol withdrawal. Treatment with typical anticonvulsants is not indicated for simple withdrawal seizures although benzodiazepines are generally given and may prevent the development of more severe withdrawal. Chronic antiseizure medication is not recommended for the prophylaxis of withdrawal seizures. An alcoholic on chronic anticonvulsive therapy is prone to withdraw from both the medication and alcohol; the result may then be status epilepticus rather than a single seizure.

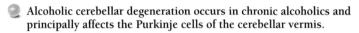 Alcoholic hallucinosis begins 1 to 2 days after the last drink. The hallucinations are not frightening and not accompanied by signs of marked autonomic stimulation.

This is the typical "pink elephant" hallucination. These last for 1 to 2 days.

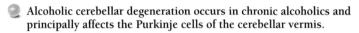 DTs typically begins 3 to 5 days after the last drink and may last as long as a week. Frightening hallucinations, disorientation, sympathetic stimulation with tachycardia, hypertension, hyperthermia, and diaphoresis dominate the clinical course.

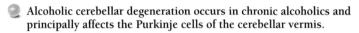 The hallucinations in DTs frequently involve images of fire.

DTs are serious and may be fatal if not treated appropriately. Benzodiazepines are the agents of choice but care to avoid oversedation is critical.

ALCOHOL AND THE HEART

The relationship between alcohol intake and heart disease is complex since it follows a "J" shaped curve: modest intake (approximately one or two drinks per day) is associated with decreased coronary artery disease and decreased all-cause mortality, while intake in excess of two or three drinks per day is associated with decreased survival. Four to five drinks per day is associated with an increase in hypertension, and serious alcoholics are at risk for alcoholic cardiomyopathy.

🫧 **Alcoholic cardiomyopathy occurs in long-standing heavy drinkers and reflects the direct toxic effects of alcohol as well as the impact of nutritional deficiencies particularly the lack of thiamine.**

The "wet" form of beriberi is a dilated cardiomyopathy with peripheral vaso-dilation and high output failure. Thiamine deficiency may contribute to the dilated cardiomyopathy that occurs in chronic alcoholics, but alcohol-induced hypertension is also a factor as is the direct toxic effect of excessive alcohol intake.

🫧 **The clinical presentation of alcoholic cardiomyopathy is usually dominated by signs of right heart failure; anasarca is not unusual and bilateral pleural effusions and ascites may be present.**

The presence of Laennec's cirrhosis may complicate the clinical picture with ascites and edema.

🫧 **All alcoholics presenting with heart failure should receive intravenous thiamine as part of the therapeutic regimen.**

🫧 **Rhythm disturbances, particularly, atrial tachycardias and atrial fibrillation are also common in patients with alcoholic cardiomyopathy.**

🫧 **The term "holiday heart" refers to arrhythmias occurring after binge drinking in patients who are not necessarily chronic alcoholics.**

Atrial fibrillation and other supraventricular tachycardias subside after the alcohol wears off.

HEMATOLOGIC CONSEQUENCES OF ALCOHOLISM

Chronic alcoholism affects all three hematologic cell lines with resultant anemia, leukopenia, and thrombocytopenia (Table 15-1). The mechanisms involved are manifold and involve direct effects of alcohol, nutritional deficiencies, concurrent Laennec's cirrhosis, and hypersplenism.

🫧 **Hypersplenism, a consequence of portal hypertension in Laennec's cirrhosis, affects all of the three cell lines singly or in any combination.**

TABLE 15.1 Hematological Consequences of Alcoholism and Laennec's Cirrhosis

Anemia

Direct toxic effect on erythroid precursors (vacuolization)

Folate deficiency (megaloblastic anemia)

Hypersplenism

Erythrocyte membrane abnormalities (spur cells, stomatocytes) → hemolysis

GI bleeding (varices, peptic ulcer disease)

Thrombocytopenia

Direct toxic effect on megakaryocytes

Hypersplenism

Neutropenia

Direct toxic effect on granulocyte precursors

Hypersplenism

Coagulopathy

Thrombocytopenia

Thrombocytopathy (impaired platelet function)

Decreased hepatic synthesis of clotting factors (cirrhosis)

Vitamin K deficiency

Scurvy (vitamin C deficiency → impaired capillary integrity)

GI blood loss from bleeding varices or from peptic ulcer disease (increased in cirrhosis) contributes to anemia as well.

Direct Toxic Effects of Alcohol

🔹 Bone marrow suppression with vacuolization of RBC, neutrophil, and platelet precursors affects the development of all three cell lines and may result in diminished levels of all the cellular elements: anemia, neutropenia, and thrombocytopenia.

Red cell development is most affected. Alcohol also may be associated with the formation of ringed sideroblasts, further contributing to suppression of red cell formation.

🔹 Alcohol and/or alcoholic liver disease induce alterations in RBC membranes that result in hemolysis.

Stomatocytes and spur cells may be seen on peripheral blood smear, abnormalities reflecting defects in the RBC membranes.

Folate Deficiency

🔹 Excessive alcohol intake is the most common cause of folate deficiency in the United States.

🔹 Poor dietary intake and impaired absorption of folate both contribute to the megaloblastic anemia frequently encountered in alcoholics.

Folate in foodstuffs is in the polyglutamate form and requires deconjugation before it can be absorbed. Alcohol is one of the several factors that impair the deconjugating enzyme.

Alcohol-induced Coagulopathy

🔹 Bleeding diatheses in alcoholics are multifactorial: thrombocytopenia, poor platelet function, and diminished synthesis of clotting factors in cirrhosis all contribute.

Prolonged prothrombin time is the clinically useful measure of hepatic synthetic function.

🔹 Vitamin K deficiency from poor dietary intake may also contribute to the bleeding diathesis and prolonged prothrombin time.

Antibiotic treatment may also contribute by diminishing the gut bacterial synthesis of vitamin K.

🔹 Vitamin C deficiency, scurvy, impairs collagen synthesis and affects capillary integrity; bleeding is a consequence, most commonly in the skin and gums.

Alcoholism is the most common cause of scurvy in the United States.

🔹 Perifollicular hemorrhages are the hallmark of scurvy.

Fatal, if untreated, scurvy rapidly responds to vitamin C administration.

Index

Note: Page number followed by f and t indicate figure and table respectively.

I took a Pill In Ibiza by
Mike Posner